JAPANESE MICHIGAN FELLOWS IN PHARMACOLOGY

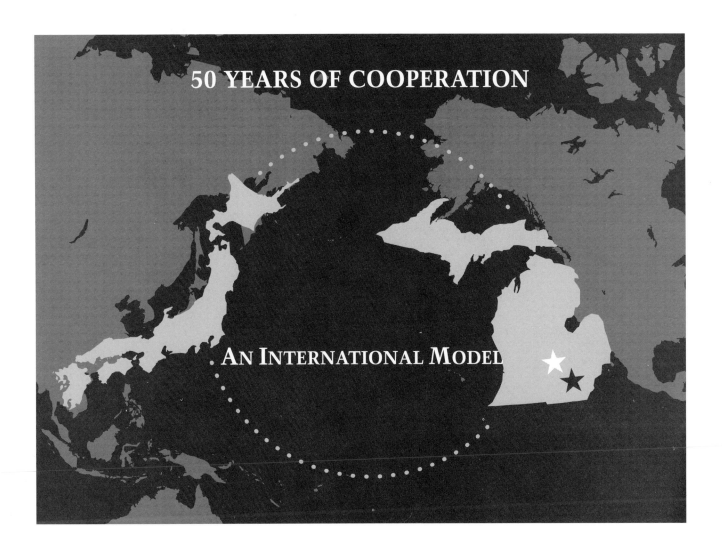

50 YEARS OF COOPERATION

AN INTERNATIONAL MODEL

Edward F. Domino, M.D.
Tomoji Yanagita, M.D., Ph.D.

Editors

NPP Books
Ann Arbor, Michigan, USA

NPP Books, Ann Arbor, MI 48106, USA
Printed in the United States of America

International Standard Book Number: 0-916182-11-8
Library of Congress Catalog Card Number: 98-68121

Acknowledgements
The efforts of Jaime E. Noce, Antoinette F. Domino, and Ellen Howard
are gratefully acknowledged.

Typeset in Palatino 12/14

∞ The paper used in this publication meets the minimum requirements of the American National Standard for Information Sciences—Permanence of Paper for Printed Library Materials, ANSI Z39.48-1984.

Dedication

This volume is dedicated to the postdoctoral fellows, their mentors, and their respective families who were, are, or will be involved in a unique Japanese and American collaboration which has existed since 1951.

Preface

◄○►

We humans are a curious lot! We have within us the capacity to hate our fellow humans enough to destroy them, and the technology to destroy our entire planet. And yet we can also be compassionate, understanding and caring for those less fortunate. The incredible suffering and loss of human life for both the victors and the vanquished during World War II are well documented. The reconstruction of the devastated postwar Japan involved many changes in various aspects of Japanese society under American influence. One of these was in medical education and care. In this complex process of regrowth, former foes became friends.

The initiatives undertaken after 1945 resulted in the remarkable nation which is Japan today. Improvements in medical education and care were a priority because Japan at that time was years behind Western nations. There was a pressing need for help. Typical of Americans, various private organizations sent medical experts to Japan in a series of medical missions.

Thus it was that one of a number of pharmacologists, Maurice Seevers, was asked to participate. Dr. Seevers specifically was asked to advise the Japanese on teaching and research on the newer medicines then available in the United States. This he did with energy, enthusiasm, and showmanship, making an incredible impression. He initiated the collection of many precious drugs as gifts from American pharmaceutical and chemical companies and their distribution in Japan. In 1951, his demonstration that a morphine-induced coma is antagonized by nalorphine astounded Japanese students, pharmacologists, and administrators alike. Young Japanese pharmacologists wanted to learn more of American pharmacological advances.

So began the story of the Seevers Michigan Fellows. This book documents the impact Michigan had on them, and their impact on those Michigan professors with whom they interacted as postdoctoral fellows in pharmacology. It should be told if to no one else then at the very least to the persons involved. This book is written especially for them. All of us have been rewarded for our interactions and cooperation. It is hoped that this program may continue into the twenty-first century. Perhaps there is a lesson to be learned for all. You, the reader, can be the judge.

March 1, 1999

Edward F. Domino
Tomogi Yanagita

SEEVERS JAPANESE MICHIGAN FELLOWS, DATES OF STAY, AND THE FACULTY LABORATORY IN WHICH THEY WORKED

No.	Name	Years of Stay	Mentor
1	Eikichi Hosoya*	1952–1954	T.M. Brody
2	Tsuneyoshi Tanabe*	1956–1957	E.J. Cafruny*
3	Showa Ueki*	1957–1959	E.F. Domino
4	Akira Sakuma	1958–1960	L. Beck
5	Kengo Nakai	1959–1960	G.A. Deneau*
6	Shuji Takaori	1959–1961	G.A. Deneau*
7	Hiroshi Kaneto	1959–1960	L.A. Woods
8	Kiro Shimamoto*	1960–1961	H.H. Swain
9	Tomoji Yanagita	1960–1965	G.A. Deneau*
10	Shiro Hisada	1961–1962	D.R. Bennett
11	Shoichi Iida	1961–1963	G.A. Deneau*
12	Tatsuo Furukawa	1961–1963	T.M. Brody
13	Tadashi Murano	1962–1963	T.M. Brody
14	Tai Akera	1962–1964	T.M. Brody
15	Nobuo Katsuda*	1963–1965	E.F. Domino
16	Reizo Inoki	1963–1965	G.A. Deneau*
17	Ken-ichi Yamamoto	1963–1965	E.F. Domino
18	Sadao Miyata	1964–1965	T.M. Brody
19	Sakutaro Tadokoro	1965–1967	J. Villarreal*
20	Akira Tsujimoto	1965–1967	R. Hudson, C.C. Hug, Jr.
21	Hiroshi Ito*	1965–1966	L. Beck
22	Matué Miyasaka*	1966–1968	E.F. Domino
23	Yoshihisa Nakai	1966–1968	E.F. Domino
24	Teiji Iwami*	1966–1968	B.R. Lucchesi
25	Kichihiko Matsusaki	1967–1968	H.H. Swain
26	Tetsuo Oka	1967–1969	C.C. Hug, Jr.
27	Fumio Ikomi	1968–1970	J.H. Woods
28	Takeo Fukuda	1968–1969	J. Villarreal*
29	Izuru Matsuoka	1968–1970	E.F. Domino
30	Toru Otani	1969–1971	H.H. Swain
31	Eiichi Hasegawa	1969–1970	C.B. Smith, T.R. Tephly
32	Naohisa Fukuda	1981–1982	E.F. Domino
33	Tsuneyuki Yamamoto	1982–1984, 1988	J.H. Woods
34	Kohji Takada	1983–1985	J.H. Woods
35	Masaru Minami	1985–1986	B.R. Lucchesi
36	Mitsuhiro Yoshioka	1989–1990	C.B. Smith
37	Shin-ichi Iwata	1993–1995	M. Gnegy
38	Toru Endo	1994–1995	C.B. Smith
39	Yuji Sudo	1994–1995	B.R. Lucchesi
40	Shiroh Kishioka	1995–1997	J.H. Woods
41	Katsuharu Saito	1996–1997	B.R. Lucchesi
42	Hiroko Togashi	1996	C.B. Smith

*Deceased

CONTENTS

————◄○►————

Section I. Overview

Section II. Early Beginnings

Section III. Japanese Seevers Postdoctoral Fellows: Michigan and Beyond Through the Years

Section IV. Other Japanese Postdoctoral Research Fellows

Section V. The University of Michigan and Japan: Present and Future Collaboration

Appendices

Section I.　Overview

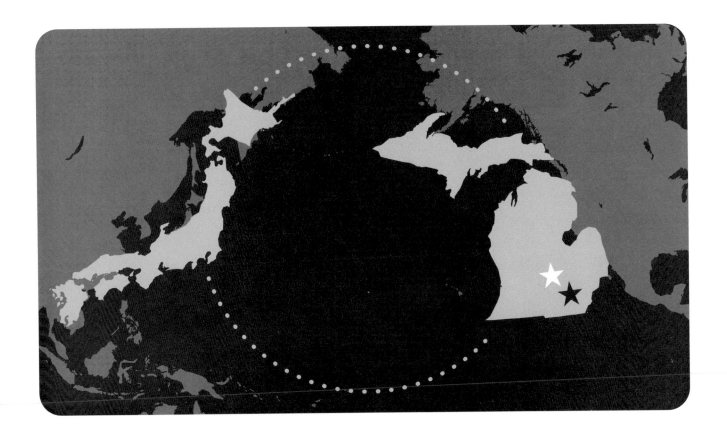

Japanese Michigan Fellows and Their Impact: A Personal Account

Edward F. Domino, M.D.

The Japanese Michigan Fellows Society exists because of the efforts of my first chairman of pharmacology at the University of Michigan, Dr. Maurice Seevers. He hired me and assigned me postdoctoral fellows from Japan to work in my laboratory. The term "Seevers Fellow" began with that assignment and others made at that time.

In early 1953, Dr. Seevers offered me a nine-month appointment as an instructor in pharmacology at the University of Michigan. I tried to get a better deal, but with Dr. Seevers it was "take it or leave it." I was never able to negotiate better terms.

Once I arrived at Dr. Seevers' office, I met Dotty Norton (later Overbeck), the whole of his departmental administration. When she went to tell Dr. Seevers I was waiting, the door had been left ajar and I could hear him say, "Dr. Domino, who?" When she reminded him he had just hired me, his response was a simple, "Oh, yeah." I knew right then and there that I had made quite an impression on him — he couldn't even remember who I was! So began my years with Dr. Seevers.

My first important research job was working with Seevers' morphine-dependent monkeys. He wanted to record the brain waves of monkeys during a cycle of morphine dependence. I was supposed to figure out how to do it.

The first Seevers Fellow to work in my laboratory at Michigan was Dr. Showa Ueki.

While he was enrolled in the English Language Institute here in Ann Arbor in 1957, Dr. Seevers decided he should be assigned to work with me. As a young assistant professor, I had little say in the matter except to agree. Those of you who knew Seevers know exactly what I mean! Although I agreed, I had considerable doubts about such an arrangement. The only Japanese with whom I had come into direct personal contact until that time was Dr. Eikichi Hosoya, who in 1953 had just been made an instructor and had been in Dr. Ted Brody's lab the year before. Thus, it came to be that both Dr. Hosoya and I were instructors at Michigan during the same period of time. He spent most of his time in Dr. Lauren Woods' laboratory on the first floor of the pharmacology building, working rather secretively on opioid research. I was on the third floor, working on a morphine project for Dr. Seevers, so Dr. Hosoya and I rarely interacted during that time except for the occasional hello. In 1956, Dr. Tsuneyoshi Tanabe came to the department, but he worked with Dr. Cafruny who was on the second floor, so I didn't interact very much with Dr. Tanabe either.

My relationship with Dr. Ueki, who came to the department a year later, was quite different. He and I worked together in the laboratory every day and night, so we got to know each other quite well. Showa completely changed my personal feelings about the

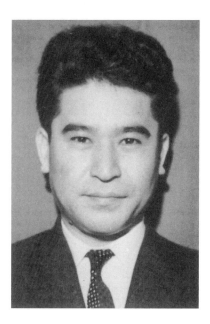

Fig. 1. A young Showa Ueki.

Japanese and their country, from wartime enemies to friends. The Japanese I have met since I first became friends with Dr. Showa Ueki have profoundly affected my life, both personally and professionally. Since that time, both Drs. Hosoya and Tanabe also became very important to me.

Showa and I were a very successful team. Almost every day we discovered something new and exciting. After we had solved the problem of implanting chronic electrodes into the brains of monkeys, we were able to study the effects of acute doses of morphine on brain wave activity.

One of our experiments, which was very interesting to me, was with a drug-naive chronic monkey given an acute dose of morphine. While the monkey was sitting in a chair and nodding just like a heroin addict, we recorded huge EEG slow waves. When I stimulated the monkey, it would become alert and its EEG would show a low-voltage desynchronization pattern. The EEG record was really beautiful. When I showed it to Dr. Seevers, he asked what it meant. I explained that after morphine the monkey was sedated and the EEG showed slow waves; when stimulated, the animal became alert and the EEG

was activated. Dr. Seevers grunted and said, "For —— sake, is that what the EEG is good for? I can look at the monkey and tell you the same thing."

Some months later, Dr. Seevers suggested I should be doing research totally on my own instead of working on his monkey project. Yet again, I must have made a wonderful impression on him, as I had that first day. I never thought I would have a future at Michigan with Dr. Seevers as the chairman.

Inasmuch as Showa and I had solved the problem of placing chronic indwelling brain electrodes in monkeys, I decided we should do the same in dogs. The problem was that mongrel dogs vary enormously in size, including in the size of their brains. Hence, we decided to use beagles. At that time, there were many beagle breeders in Michigan, so I was able to obtain from them rejected dogs who were either too old, infertile, or had psychological problems such as excessive nervousness or just plain craziness. Instead of the breeders euthanizing these dogs, I was able to obtain them almost for free, paying primarily for their transportation. (Incidentally, in recent years, Dr. Ben Lucchesi in our department reinstated such an arrangement for his own cardiovascular research.)

Showa and I had to first prepare our own atlas of the beagle brain in stereotaxic coordinates. This we did, and I planned to publish it someday. In 1959, Adrianov and Mering published in Russian *An Atlas of the Canine Brain*, which I decided should be translated into English. Eventually, I got the English version published in 1964. In the process, my wife and I learned how to publish books.

One day, Showa and I were doing an EEG study with one of our crazy chronic beagles. The dog, very excited, kept moving excessively in its Pavlov frame. All we could record was skeletal muscle artifacts. I asked Showa to try to calm the dog, so he went into our shielded, sound-proof room where the dog was and shut the door. After a few minutes of recording nothing but movement artifact, all of a sudden the artifacts ceased. A low-voltage activated EEG pattern appeared in the neocortex and incredible high-voltage synchronous waves appeared in the amygdala. Astounded, I ran to the door and opened it, asking Showa what had happened. He was smoking a cigarette; in those days, the University buildings were not "smoke-free," as they are today. Showa explained that he had decided to smoke a cigarette and to blow smoke into the animal's nose; he had noted on a previous occasion that tobacco smoke would quiet this dog. Showa and I didn't know it at the time, but in the past 10 years there have been a lot of data that nicotine and tobacco smoke improve sensory gating of irrelevant stimuli in human schizophrenic patients, though only transiently. So it was in our very agitated dog; the calming effects lasted only a short time.

Inasmuch as Dr. Seevers permitted me to apply for my own research grants, I immediately decided to find a private granting agency interested in tobacco smoke, since National Institute of Health money was not available. I applied and received a grant from the Council for Tobacco Research to further study this interesting phenomenon. Thanks to Showa Ueki, I've been involved in nicotine and tobacco research ever since. It turned out that all kinds of smoke activate the amygdala and olfactory bulb. This led me in two different directions: olfaction research and nicotine research.

Showa and I first pursued the role of smoke and different smells on olfactory bulb and limbic activity in the dog. Showa designed a super air purifier system and showed that absolutely pure air without any odors causes a burst of electrical activity which enhances the effect of an odor. We discovered the physiological basis of sniffing. When we wrote up our findings to be published in the prestigious *Journal of Neurophysiology*, the peer reviewers were extremely critical, but eventually, after further research, our work was published in that journal. Since that time, no one ever refers to our "classic" paper, but you, the reader, now know the reason people sniff when smelling an odor.

I knew at that time that Eccles and his associates in Australia had shown that the Golgi recurrent collateral-Renshaw inhibitory neuron synapse in the spinal cord was mediated by acetylcholine. Was it muscarinic or nicotinic? I thought it was the latter and decided we should study this synapse in the spinal cord. This meant becoming experts in microelectrode techniques. Neither Showa nor I was good at it. When I heard that Dr. K. Koketsu, who had studied with Eccles, was at the University of Illinois in Chicago, I contacted him and proposed that Showa be trained in his laboratory. He agreed, so Showa went to Chicago and learned microelectrode techniques. All three of us published our results with mecamylamine, a ganglionic-blocking agent which penetrates the blood-brain barrier. Clearly the spinal cord synapse activated by acetylcholine and nicotine is a nicotinic cholinergic synapse. Later, Koketsu became a famous professor of physiology in Japan.

Showa returned to Fukuoka in 1959, and four years later Dr. Seevers assigned Dr. Nobuo Katsuda to me. He also was from Fukuoka. Dr. Katsuda was skilled in electrophysiology and brought with him knowledge of techniques that I did not possess. In fact, over the years I've been very poor at using microelectrode techniques. In my own personal experiments, I would get my best recordings from midnight on, which grossly messed up my wife's and my sleep schedule. Dr. Katsuda was interested in the relationship between evoked potentials and single unit recordings using mice. He insisted that mice work best because the famous Spanish neuroanatomist, Ramon de Cajal, showed that the mouse neocortex contains a simplified but basic architecture of the human neocortex. Therefore, a simplified neuronal system would be the best to study. Dr. Katsuda spent many long and tedious hours collecting a

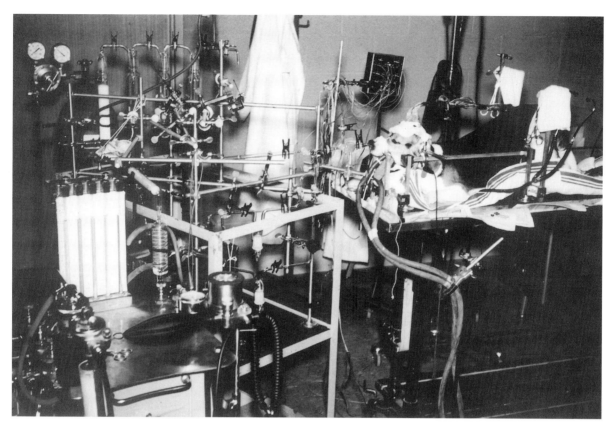

Fig. 2. One of Dr. S. Ueki's canine subjects under balanced general anesthesia. The photograph shows the complex experimental setup for recording electrical activity in olfactory and limbic brain structures to various odors and ultrapure air.

great deal of data. I decided that it was not as interesting to me as to him and suggested he publish his findings in Japanese.

When he returned to Japan, he did very well, as did Showa. Dr. Katsuda became a professor of pharmacology in the dental faculty, and Dr. Ueki was a professor of pharmacology in the pharmacy faculty, both at Kyushu University in Fukuoka. Showa was a great storyteller and Katsuda a great listener. Both had such unique personal skills that they did very well back home in Japan.

There is one more story about Seevers and Ueki which I must tell. Dr. Seevers drove an old automobile that was in very bad shape. One day, he offered it to Showa for free. In those days, a car to the Japanese was something very precious, so of course Showa accepted before he had a chance to drive it. I told Showa that Seevers' car was junk, which he shouldn't have taken, even for nothing. Showa ignored my advice and was very

proud of that "junk." Subsequently, as Ueki and his family toured Michigan and then the United States, they had major repair problems. Showa spent most of his fellowship

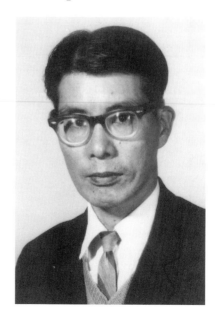

Fig. 3. Nobuo Katsuda while in my lab.

money repairing that car, but still he told many stories about his "wonderful free car" that Seevers had given him. I assume that all he and his family ate while living in Ann Arbor was rice, in order to pay the bills created by that piece of junk.

Dr. Ken-ichi Yamamoto also arrived in my laboratory in 1963. He had previously been working at the Shionogi Pharmaceutical Company in Osaka, and had a lot of experience with indwelling brain electrodes in cats and the EEG effects of various drugs. Since his interest completely overlapped with mine, it was logical that he study the EEG effects of nicotine in more detail. This he did very well and soon had excellent data on the effects of nicotine on the awake-sleep cycle of the cat. We published a great deal of interesting data indicating nicotine had a clear wake-up effect and activated the EEG of a sleeping cat. Subsequently, the amount of REM sleep increased. Lysine vasopressin also increased REM sleep so we thought the nicotine REM effect was due to vasopressin release. Years later, I tried to show that subcutaneous nicotine at bedtime increased REM sleep in a few humans but was unable to do so. However, the interaction of vasopressin and REM sleep is still a worthy area of pursuit because the cat data was very convincing. Scientifically, Ken-ichi and I worked well and productively together.

Dr. Yamamoto returned to Japan in 1965. That year, as part of the XXIIIrd International Congress of Physiological Sciences in Japan, Professor T. Tokizane of Tokyo University Faculty of Medicine held a satellite meeting in Hakone. Inasmuch as Ken-ichi had previously trained with Professor Tokizane, it was no surprise that I was invited to that satellite, which was for me an enormous scientific success. In addition, it was the first trip which my wife, Toni, and I made to Japan. Fortunately, Toni's mother stayed in Ann Arbor with our young children so that she could go with me to Japan. From Detroit we flew to Chicago, and there boarded a charter flight to Tokyo via Anchorage, Alaska. Our first trip to Japan!

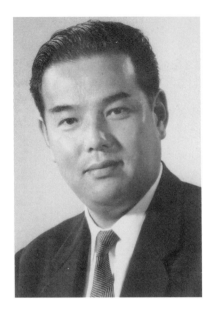

Fig. 4. A youthful Ken-ichi Yamamoto.

How can we express in words our many memorable experiences? We were treated as real VIPs, staying at the old Imperial Hotel in Tokyo, which had been designed by Frank Lloyd Wright, before it was razed. It was replaced by the new Imperial, which years later we always visit, though we were never able to afford to stay there. We also went to Nikko, Hakone, and Osaka. In each city, we got the royal treatment, as only the Japanese can provide. On this trip, I brought with me a computer of average transients which the electronic engineers at Shionogi marveled at, took

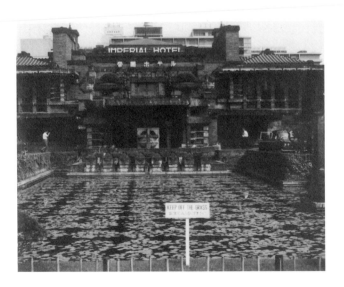

Fig. 5. The Imperial Hotel, Tokyo, 1965.

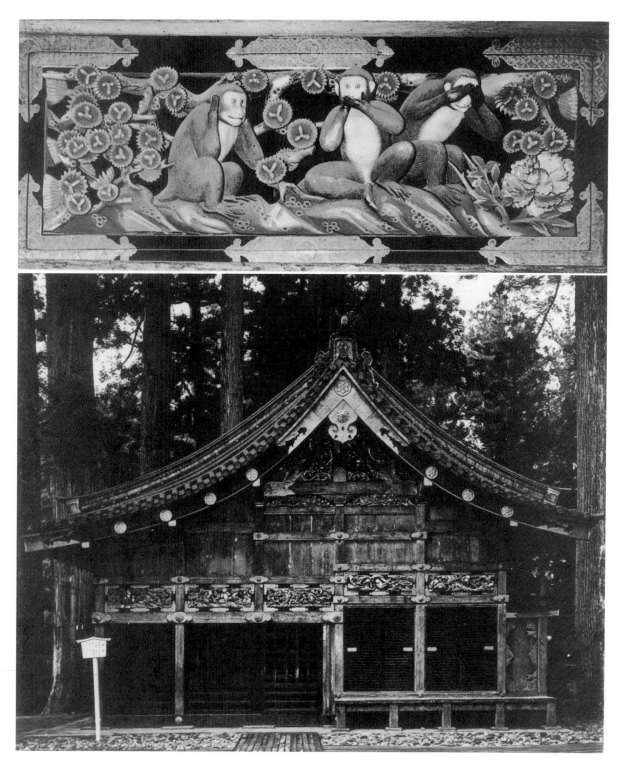

Fig. 6. Nikko's famous three monkeys at the Toshogu Shrine above the door of the Sacred Stable, 1965. Hear no evil, speak no evil, see no evil.

apart, and put back together, without schematic drawings.

While in Osaka, we had an encounter with a typhoon that destroyed a portion of the railroad track between Kyoto and Tokyo. It nearly caused us to miss our charter flight home from Tokyo. Thanks to Ken-ichi, we made it back to Tokyo by plane. During this first trip to Japan, Toni and I learned about Kobe beef and Sapporo, Kirin, and Asahi beer.

The yen/dollar exchange rate was grossly in favor of the dollar. An expensive Kobe steak meal seemed to us incredibly cheap. Furthermore, each of us had a personal white gloved waiter who anticipated our every gastronomic need. We never experienced such attention before or since. Also during this trip, Toni became a connoisseur of Japanese beers and sake — all in moderation of course. She still feels Kirin is best. I prefer Sapporo beer.

In 1966, Drs. Matué Miyasaka and Yoshihisa Nakai joined my laboratory in Ann Arbor. Since Matué was interested in EEG research, I involved him in a project on ketamine. Yoshihisa, on the other hand, with his background in microelectrode research in Kyoto, did more basic studies. When Matué returned to Japan, he subsequently became professor of neuropsychiatry at Dokkyo University and Yoshihisa set up a private clinic, the Nakai Clinic. Izuru Matsuoka arrived in 1968 to conduct microelectrode research, and Naohisa Fukuda from Takeda Pharmaceutical Company came in 1981 to do EEG studies in monkeys. Izuru became an otolaryngologist in clinical practice, while Naohisa returned to Takeda; both are in Osaka.

Hence, I've had seven official Japanese

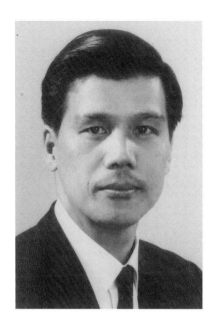

Fig. 8. Yoshihisa Nakai looking thoughtful.

fellows in my laboratory, who have made many contributions to our knowledge of pharmacology. They helped move my own research endeavors into areas which I alone could not have accomplished. My interactions with the official Japanese fellows was so rewarding, I decided to obtain other fellows from Japan directly, outside of the formal Seevers program (see Chapter 17).

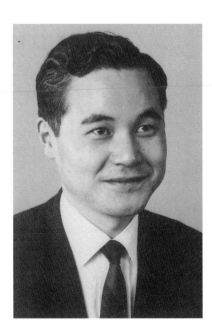

Fig. 7. Matué Miyasaka smiling, as usual.

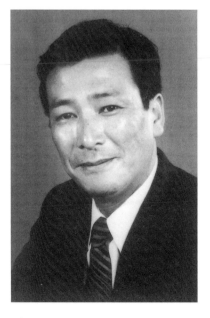

Fig. 9. A pleased Izuru Matsuoka.

2

The Japanese Pharmacologists Who Came to Michigan

Henry H. Swain, M.D.

In 1954 I was appointed to the faculty of the University of Michigan Department of Pharmacology where Japanese pharmacologists soon became an important part of my life. In 1951 the departmental chairman, Dr. M.H. Seevers, had visited Japan as a member of the Second U.S. Medical Mission. Soon after his return, pharmacologists whom he had met in Japan began to come to Ann Arbor. Some stayed only a few days, some visited for several weeks, and many remained at the University of Michigan for a year or more.

The impact of Japanese pharmacologists upon my life began with a visit from a man whom I met only briefly. A few months after I joined the department, Dr. Seevers brought to my laboratory a visitor from Nagasaki. Professor Y. Nakazawa was traveling in the United States and came to Ann Arbor to see Dr. Seevers. Dr. Nakazawa brought with him a manuscript, soon to be published in the *Japanese Journal of Pharmacology,* which had been written by two of his colleagues in the Department of Pharmacology at the Nagasaki University School of Medicine. It was entitled "A New Measurement of Blood Flow," and its authors were Drs. Akira Ueno and Fumio Takenaka.

The manuscript described an ingenious rolling, mercury-filled manometer, capable of measuring the difference between the pressure exerted by the blood before and after it passes through an orifice or a constriction.

The pressure difference is related to the rate at which the blood is flowing. This manometer made it easy to record changes in blood flow on a smoked-paper kymograph, which was a common recording device in the pharmacology laboratories of 50 years ago. After reading the manuscript which Dr. Nakazawa had brought, I was very interested and decided immediately to build a manometer like the one described by Drs. Ueno and Takenaka. My manometer worked so well that we used it both as a research tool and as a teaching device for our medical students. I described it in a short article which I published in the *University of Michigan Medical Bulletin.*

Because of that short article, I received a brief moment of unexpected (and undeserved) fame. My name appeared in *TIME* magazine! In the issue of February 6, 1956, *TIME* ran a very short paragraph, as one of several items under the heading of "New Medical Wrinkles":

A cheap, simple meter to measure blood flow directly. It was made by Dr. Henry H. Swain of the University of Michigan from the pinion gear of a discarded alarm clock, stiff wire, rubber tubing, [and] glass bulbs. The tube is inserted directly into an artery. Blood passes through the tube, [and] moves a pen that records on a graph any changes in blood flow. Cost $10.

11

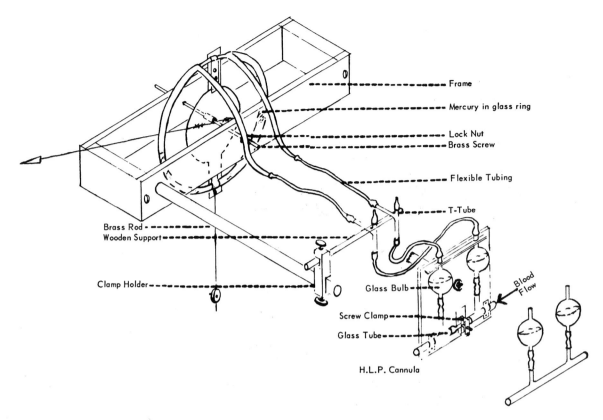

Fig. 1. Flowmeter modeled after Drs. Ueno and Takenaka.

I do not know why this little article appeared in *TIME*. The flow meter might be useful to people working in laboratories, but it is not important enough to justify publication in a famous national magazine. Perhaps some editor was amused by the thought of a person making something useful from a discarded alarm clock. However it happened, that little article was noticed by many of my friends, and I kept receiving congratulations for months after that.

Dr. Seevers was angry about the little article in *TIME* because it did not mention the Japanese pharmacologists who had made the original invention. To him it looked as if I had stolen the idea of Drs. Ueno and Takenaka and had not given them the proper credit. However, in the article which I wrote for the *University of Michigan Medical Bulletin*, I acknowledged Drs. Ueno, Takenaka, and also Nakazawa quite properly. I cannot accept responsibility for the author of the *TIME* article, someone who apparently did not even understand how the flow meter works.

I am grateful to Drs. Nakazawa, Ueno, and Takenaka for making me famous in the eyes of my friends who read *TIME*, even though I did get scolded by Dr. Seevers. Many years after the flow-meter adventure, Dr. Ueno came to Ann Arbor and served for a

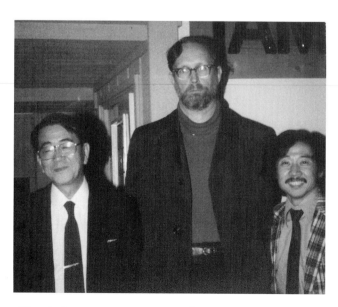

Fig. 2. Drs. Ueno, Swain, and T. Yamamoto, 1982.

year as a visiting professor of pharmacology at the University of Michigan. He was also present at the Centennial Celebration in 1991.

Another Japanese pharmacologist who contributed to my professional development was Dr. Shuji Takaori from Kyoto. From 1959 to 1961 Dr. Takaori served as a postdoctoral fellow. For a short time before joining the laboratory of Dr. Deneau, he worked with Dr. Lloyd Beck. Dr. Beck and I worked independently of one another but our laboratories were in one large room. Therefore Dr. Beck's students and my students interacted with one another almost every day. I discovered that Dr. Takaori had recently published a very interesting observation concerning the effect of EDTA (ethylenediamine tetra-acetic acid, the calcium ion chelator) on the shape of the action potential from heart muscle. Soon we had set up our own micro-electrode experiments. We had no difficulty reproducing Dr. Takaori's findings, and I spent many months attempting to use this observation to explain the origin of certain abnormal heart rhythms.

Dr. Tomoji Yanagita, whose first appointment in Ann Arbor was from 1960 to 1965, designed and built for me an electronic model to show how impulses are conducted in heart muscle. It consisted of five brick-sized boxes, each of which represented an excitable cell, complete with a threshold for excitation, an absolute refractory period, a relative refractory period, and the ability to deliver a stimulus to a neighboring cell. The five excitable cells were connected in a ring and could demonstrate a "circus rhythm", such as is thought to exist in heart muscle which is in a state of flutter or fibrillation. The Yanagita model was so successful that my students and I moved on to a simulation of fibrillation on a digital computer, a project that eventually provided two young men with their doctoral dissertations in the field of Computer and Communication Sciences.

Life in the pharmacology laboratory was not all work; there was also some play. In my case, play was the game of GO. My first teacher of GO was Dr. Akira Sakuma, who was a fellow in Dr. Beck's laboratory from 1958 to 1960. My more advanced training came from Dr. Kiro Shimamoto, a *shodan* who was in my laboratory in 1961 and 1962. (Dr. Shimamoto taught me how to play GO and in return, I taught him about "echo beats" in the heart.) There was a GO club in Ann Arbor in those days, and in the evenings, Dr. Shimamoto and I would attend its meetings. My GO playing continued with Dr. Kichihiko Matsusaki, who studied in my laboratory in 1967 and 1968, and with Dr. Toru Otani, who was with me in 1970 and 1971.

The high moment of my GO playing occurred not in Michigan but in Japan. One of the brief visitors to the department was Dr. Y. Aramaki. During his visit, he and I sat in the office of Dr. Seevers' famous monkey colony and played a game of GO. Dr. Aramaki was a much stronger player than I am, and he beat me by a large margin. In 1970, when I was visiting Japan, I again met Dr. Aramaki, and we played another game of GO. In that second game I got lucky and was able to capture a large group of stones in the center of the board. For the rest of that trip, wherever I went in Japan, my hosts would greet me by saying with admiration, "You beat Dr. Ara-

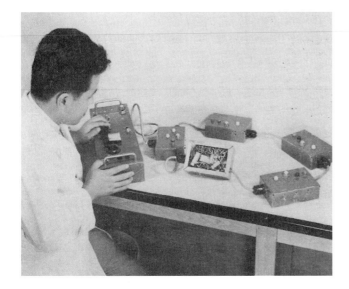

Fig. 3. Dr. Yanagita with the electronic model he built for Dr. Swain.

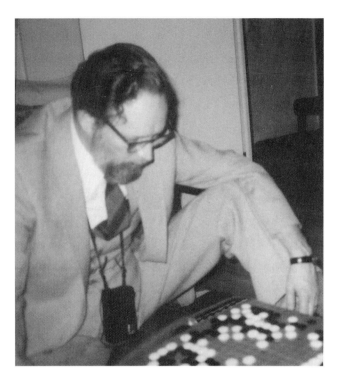

Fig. 4. Dr. Swain in deep concentration.

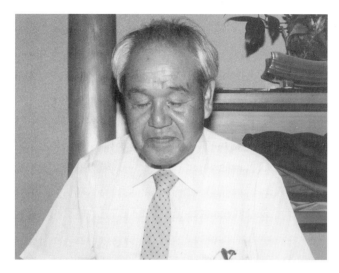

Fig. 5. Dr. Matsusaki meditating.

maki at GO!" The "grapevine" among Japanese pharmacologists is wonderful.

Golf is another game which I shared with some of my Japanese colleagues. (Golf is so much cheaper to play in the United States than it is in Japan, that those people who liked the game could hardly resist the temptation to play while they were here.) Dr. Yanagita and I often played the small course called "Pat's Par 3", which used to be just east of Ann Arbor. Dr. Matsusaki and Dr. Otani both played the Radrick Farms course with me. However, the best of the golf games as far as I'm concerned was hosted by Dr. Otani when Dr. Edward Cafruny and I were visiting Sapporo in 1986.

When Japanese visitors were in Ann Arbor, we tried to make them feel welcome. Dr. and Mrs. Seevers were particularly skillful at such entertainment, and we other faculty members held parties occasionally. The social efforts which we made in Ann Arbor were repaid many, many times over when any of us subsequently visited Japan.

In 1970 there was a World's Fair in

Osaka — EXPO '70. Twenty-five years before (1945–1946) I had lived in Osaka, and so I decided to take my wife, Vicki, and two teen-aged children with me to the fair. By that time I knew at least one pharmacologist in almost every major city in Japan. The hospitality which we received was fantastic. We spent 21 days in Japan and were entertained at 23 parties during that time. We went as far south as Kagoshima and as far north as Nikko. We traveled by airplane, ship, train (including the *Shin-kan-sen*), and automobile. We stayed in luxury hotels, in modest hotels, and in a *ryokan*.

In Nagasaki, Dr. Ueno introduced us to his colleague's teen-aged daughter, Masako Hongo. She speaks excellent English and served as hostess to my wife and children while I visited the Medical School. Ever since that visit we have remained in contact with Miss Hongo, who has gone on to become a famous flower arranger in Japan.

My son, David, is a professional musician. The very first time that he was paid money for performing music in public was when he was 16 years old, and it happened at EXPO '70. When we arrived in Osaka, David looked at the program of events scheduled for the next day at the fair. He found that a Japanese rock-and-roll group would be performing at the San Francisco Pavilion. We arrived at the Pavilion just as the group members were beginning to set up their heavy equipment on the stage. David helped the musicians carry their amplifiers, speakers, etc. to where they would be needed for the performance. Then the leader of the group, who spoke a little English, asked David, "Do you play guitar?" David said, "yes", and so he was invited to join the band! One of their guitar players had failed to come to the performance, and so David replaced him. For his services, David was paid 500 yen, which in those days was equivalent to about $1.50. Not a great deal of money, but it was the start of a profession. Far more important than the money was the fact the leader of the group escorted David around Osaka for the next two days, taking him home to meet his mother and have lunch, and visiting music stores and other places of their mutual interest. For David, it was the high point of his trip to Japan.

I returned to Japan in 1981 for the IUPHAR meeting in Tokyo, where again I was treated royally, particularly by Dr. Eikichi Hosoya. Dr. Hosoya was on the faculty of the University of Michigan before I was! In 1952 he became the first of a long line of Michigan scholars. At that time he was the chairman of the Department of Pharmacology at Keio University in Tokyo. For the 1952–1953 year he was a postdoctoral fellow at Michigan, and the following year he held the rank of instructor in the department. He had returned to Keio University shortly before I arrived in Ann Arbor.

Dr. Tsuneyoshi Tanabe became the second Michigan scholar, when he was appointed as an instructor in pharmacology at Michigan for the 1956–1957 year; in Japan he served for many years as a professor of pharmacology at the Hokkaido University in Sapporo. In 1986 Dr. Tanabe invited me to participate in a symposium in Sapporo. While I was there I also gave a small seminar in which I demonstrated the behavior of our computer simulation of fibrillation in heart muscle. The

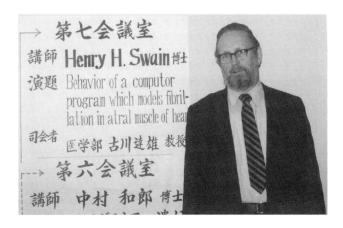

Fig. 6. Dr. Swain in Japan in 1986 with a poster of his seminar on a computer simulation model of atrial fibrillation.

man who ran the slide projector for me on that occasion was Dr. Mitsuhiro Yoshioka, who later (1989–1990) became the fourth M.H. Seevers International Fellow in Pharmacology at the University of Michigan. Even more recently, Dr. Yoshioka has been named chairman of pharmacology at the University of Hokkaido, succeeding Dr. Hideya Saito who had followed Dr. Tanabe in that chair.

In September 1991, eight Japanese pharmacologists came to Ann Arbor for our Centennial Celebration. That three-day meeting marked the 100th anniversary of the establishment of a department of pharmacology in an American university. Dr. John Jacob Abel,

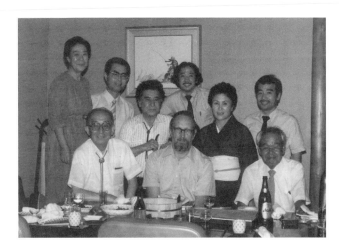

Fig. 7. A group meeting with pharmacologists in Fukuoka in 1986.

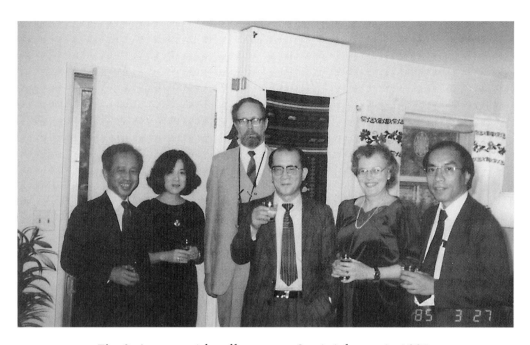

Fig. 8. A party with colleagues at Swain's house in 1985.

Michigan's first pharmacologist, had been appointed to the faculty in January 1891. We were joined in our celebration by Drs. Saito, Tsujimoto, Ueno, Yanagita, and Yoshioka, and also by Dr. Reizo Inoki (who had been in Ann Arbor during the years 1963–1965), Dr. Tetsuo Oka (1967–1969), and Dr. Kazuko Nonaka.

During the early years of Michigan scholars coming to Ann Arbor, financial support came largely from the Miles Laboratories in Elkhart, Indiana, through the generosity of Dr. Walter Compton. After Dr. Seevers died in 1977, I took the responsibility of organizing the Seevers International Fellowship in Pharmacology. Admirers of Dr. Seevers from around the world agreed that such a fellowship would be a most appropriate memorial to a man who had spent his professional life

making it possible for people to get graduate training in pharmacology. Japanese pharmacologists, led by Dr. Yanagita, were major contributors to the Seevers Fund. To date, six people have been awarded the Seevers Fellowship: Dr. Jesus Andres Garcia-Sevilla (1979–1981), Dr. Tsuneyuki Yamamoto (1982–1984), Dr. Kohji Takada (1983–1985), Dr. Mitsuhiro Yoshioka (1989–1990), Dr. Shin-ichi Iwata (1993–1995), and Dr. Shiroh Kishioka (1995–1997). At the time that the Fellowship Fund was established, it was hoped that it would continue to be active during the professional lifetimes of people who had known and worked with Dr. Seevers. However, that period of time is now drawing to an end, and a new generation is left to maintain it.

Section II.   Early Beginnings

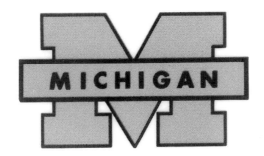

3

The Contribution of Dr. Maurice H. Seevers to Postwar Progress in Japanese Pharmacology, Beginning in 1951

Tsuneyoshi Tanabe, M.D., Ph.D.

In the late 19th century, Professor Dr. Juntaro Takahashi of the University of Tokyo Faculty of Medicine was sent to Germany to study pharmacology in the laboratory of Dr. Oswald Schmiedeberg of the University of Strassburg. Upon returning to Tokyo, he was appointed the chairman of Japan's first Department of Pharmacology at Tokyo University. His two talented pupils, Dr. Kurata Morishima and Dr. Haruo Hayashi, also studied abroad at the laboratory of Dr. Schmiedeberg. While in the German's laboratory, Professor Hayashi was a contemporary of G.N. Richards of Pennsylvania and George Wallace of New York.

Dr. Morishima was later appointed chairman of pharmacology at the Kyoto University School of Medicine. Dr. Hayashi was sent to the Kyushu University Faculty of Medicine to open the Department of Pharmacology. A few years later, he was called back to the University of Tokyo to chair the Second Department of Pharmacology in the Faculty of Medicine. Drs. Hayashi and Morishima trained many pharmacologists in their respective laboratories. These pharmacologists, in turn, spread out among the various medical schools that were newly established in numerous districts around Japan after World War I.

In those days, most medical school professors would study abroad in Europe, especially in Germany, for two years or more, except for a few who studied in England or the United States. Consequently, the German language became an indispensable subject for premedical students, and technical textbooks written in German were recommended by the medical professors. In short, medical science in Japan as taught up to World War II closely followed the German style.

As the years went by, young Japanese doctors started to become interested in the theses and monographs published in the United States. Medical textbooks written in Japanese also began to be published. However, when World War II broke out, it was not possible to obtain up-to-date scientific information from other countries. In addition, young staff members and researchers who held medical licenses were called into military service. Laboratory work at the medical schools declined markedly because unlicensed persons were not allowed to work in medical laboratories.

In the post-World War II period, beginning in 1945, physicians discharged from the military returned to their respective laboratories. However, they found it hard to get over their loss of spirit and to continue laboratory work. The importation of drugs and other materials from abroad was restricted and budgets were too small to replace aging equipment with up-to-date items. What was worse, there were severe shortages of energy resources and foodstuffs. As a result, most researchers were compelled to quit their laboratories and return to their home towns where

19

they could earn larger incomes as physicians. Nonetheless, a small group of staff members remained in most Japanese medical school departments, enduring many hardships and seeking new paths to revive activity in their universities. Their first priority became to find opportunities to study abroad in the United States. For that purpose, many began to improve their English, particularly speaking and understanding the language.

Around 1950, the Garioa and Fulbright Programs were opened for promising young scientists in Japan. At that time, the First U.S. Medical Mission was also sent to Japan.

In May, 1951, the Second U.S. Medical Mission visited Japan. Dr. Maurice Harrison Seevers, chairman of the Department of Pharmacology at the University of Michigan Medical School, was a member of this second mission. The mission members were met at Haneda Airport by Colonel Johnson of the U.S. General Headquarters and Miss Snavely (the mission's secretary). They departed for the Dai-Ichi Hotel in an Army bus. The hotel was entirely filled with American Occupation personnel, so the members of the mission could stay there at ease among their countrymen.

The mission members first met Dr. Kusama, professor of public health at Keio University School of Medicine. He was president of the Japanese Medical Society and had been Stanford-trained, making him one of the few American university graduates in Japan. He was backed by the Supreme Commander of the Allied Powers because of his knowledge of English and American methods. Dr. Kusama described current medical education in Japan to the mission members. After this discussion, the itinerary of the mission was laid out as follows:

University of Tokyo, Tokyo　　　May 14–25
Hyogo University, Kobe　　May 28–June 8
Hokkaido University, Sapporo　June 11–22.

They then went to the headquarters of the Public Health and Welfare (PH&W) sec-

tion to look at the awe-inspiring supply of drugs and chemicals which Dr. Seevers had obtained from the pharmaceutical industry prior to his departure from Michigan. The total value (tax-free) of the drugs and chemicals was between $5,000 and $10,000. At that time, this amount was considered an unbelievable sum of money. Dr. Seevers sorted out all of the drugs and chemicals and presented them to the main medical schools in Japan. Each package included invaluable compounds which were very difficult to obtain at that time in Japan and indispensable to pharmacologists.

Dr. Seevers made frequent visits to the University of Tokyo Faculty of Medicine to meet with Dean Kodama and Professor Kobayashi, chairman of the Department of Pharmacology, to arrange an educational program for a two week period. Dr. Kobayashi introduced Dr. Seevers to an interpreter, Dr. Eikichi Hosoya, assistant professor of pharmacology at Keio University, as well as other professors of pharmacology from the Tokyo area. At an introductory affair, they had green tea for about 15 minutes and then Dr. Seevers was ceremoniously presented a key to a nice office for use during his stay in Tokyo. In the evening, the Japanese Minister of Education hosted a party in a beautiful restaurant in Ueno Park for the mission members. The party was attended by university presidents, many professors emeriti, deans, and dignitaries representing the ministry and military. Dr. Seevers was greatly honored by a visit from Professor Emeritus Hayashi at the University of Tokyo; he described the latter as "a fine-appearing elderly gentleman of 77 with a beautiful handlebar mustache."

At about 9:00 A.M. the morning after the party, Dr. Seevers went to his temporary office in the Department of Pharmacology and discussed his lectures with Dr. Hosoya and Dr. Kobayashi. For his first lecture, Dr. Seevers talked on "Morphine and the Newer Synthetics" for one and a half hours to a class of 130 students and a large number of faculty mem-

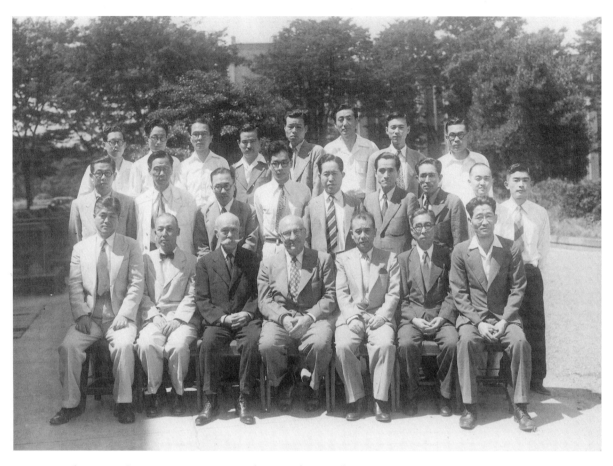

Fig. 1. Group photograph June 27, 1951 in Tokyo. Left to right - First row, E. Hosoya, M. Osawa, H. Hayashi, M. Seevers, Y. Kobayashi, H. Kumagai, K. Uraguchi. Second row, K. Hashimoto, S. Ohashi, K. Tokita, S. Takeuchi, T. Bando, H. Ito, Y. Aramaki, H. Takayanagi, A. Oga. Third row, K. Fujita, Y. Wada, S. Ebashi, H. Nukada, S. Iwasaki, S. Mori, T. Shigei, T. Yui.

bers and others from the surrounding environs. He was instructed to talk slowly so that the students could understand him, and his interpreter summarized his lectures every five minutes or so. He later joked in a letter to his family, "I only saw one kid sleeping during the whole period of my lecture which is an accomplishment!" He added that the other attending students were interested in his lecture.

The next day, the mission members spent the morning in the clinical wards of several university hospitals. Dr. Lucia, a physician, and others from the mission concluded:

1) The central dietary kitchens were incredibly dirty by American standards.
2) The Japanese concept of sterility was amusing, as the operating room floors were kept wet and personnel put on wooden *"geta"* (elevated wooden sandals) upon entering.
3) General anesthesia did not exist - they saw "a poor devil" having a cholecystectomy under a "spinal" who was moving his feet and emitting terrible groans whenever the professor of surgery probed or manipulated the abdominal contents.
4) The nurses were not exposed to higher nursing education designed to take them to the level of supervisors.

Dr. Seevers' impression was that pharmacology in Japan was at the level at which Americans had been 20 years earlier, except for the addition of some new agents. Equip-

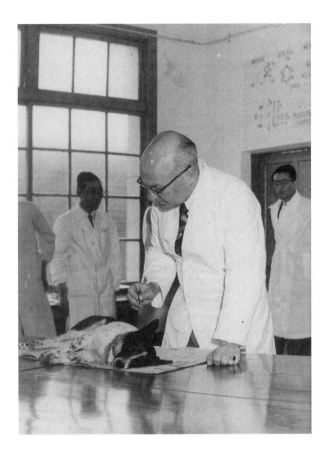

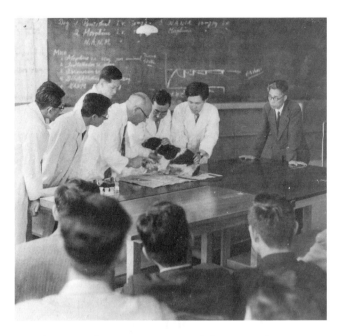

Figs. 2 and 3. May 1951 in Tokyo. Dr. Seevers demonstrating the antagonistic effect of nalorphine at the Tokyo University Faculty of Medicine. Left-a morphinized dog. Right-recovery from morphine anesthesia after nalorphine. Dr. Kumagai is at the far right. Students are in the foreground.

ment was of the old German style, even in Tokyo, which had the best and largest institutions in Japan.

On May 24, Dr. Seevers had a joint conference with the staff of the University of Tokyo to discuss American research, in general, as well as that of individual researchers. The pharmacology group from the entire Tokyo area gave a special luncheon for Dr. Seevers, at which many speeches of thanks were given by the leaders of Japanese pharmacology. The refreshments included sandwiches, specially prepared "soba" noodles, and Japanese beer. Numerous gifts were given to Dr. Seevers including his portrait which was painted in watercolor by an expert amateur who was also a professor of pharmacology at a private medical college. The most beautiful gift was a maroon cloisonné vase with a lovely flower design which was worth about 100,000 yen ($300 at that time), a small fortune for the Japanese. It was a gorgeous

item presented collectively by all members of the pharmacology departments in the Tokyo area.

In the afternoon, the Tokyo group held a party for Dr. Seevers in the beautiful library of the University of Tokyo. The library had been donated by the Rockefeller Foundation in 1926 after the great Tokyo earthquake and fire. The party finished with warm farewells accompanied by a sumptuous feast with sake, beer, and "the works." All present enjoyed a close, intimate feeling of friendship.

The next day, the mission members went to the Union Club of Tokyo where they threw a party for the Minister of Education, the presidents of the various universities, the deans, their counterparts, and the interpreters. It was a gala occasion with everybody consuming large quantities of liquor and hors d'oeuvres. After the party, Dr. Seevers and the other members left Tokyo at 10:15 P.M. by private cars provided by the Allied Forces and arrived in Nagoya at 6:00 A.M. They changed to a train for Toba and Kashikojima where they boarded Mr. Mikimoto's launch, which took them to a famous pearl farm to see the oyster seeding facility.

The next morning, they divided into four groups: the Kyoto group (Darrow, Soule, and Davidson), the Fukuoka group (Valputs, Johnson, Handler, and Snavely), the Osaka group (Lucia, Price, and Ackerman), and the Kobe group (Seevers, Beeson, and Newell). At 8:00 A.M., Dr. Seevers' group arrived at Sannomiya Station where they were met by Lt. Colonel Water and others. They were treated as real VIPs in Kobe. Their very lush hotel, called the Koshien at that time, had been patterned after a Frank Lloyd Wright design. The Commanding General of Southern Japan, who was stationed in Osaka, lived right above the big room occupied by Drs. Seevers and Beeson.

On Monday, May 28, 1951, Dr. Seevers went to the Hyogo Prefectural Medical School and met Dr. Shoji, who had come to Hyogo to run the new medical school, having retired at 60 from Kyoto University. He was a physiologist who in 1928 had studied at the University of Michigan in Ann Arbor. The Medical School building and the 500-bed hospital had been rebuilt after the bombing. Dr. Seevers' first impression was that "the floors of the building were not kept clean. The Japanese had a lot to learn about cleanliness; personally they seemed to be quite clean although their clothing might be soiled. Soap for washing clothes was costly as was labor for general cleaning in relation to the individual income of even the middle class." On Wednesday, June 6th, after a conference with the entire Osaka group, Dr. Seevers gave two lectures and a demonstration concerning his research on morphine and nalorphine. On Thursday, June 7th, two more lectures were given in the morning. Then, Dr. Seevers and two other mission members were taken to the Maiko Villa about 20 miles west of Kobe for lunch, after which they gave lectures to about 100 members of the Kobe Medical Association.

On Saturday, Dr. Seevers and the others arrived at Haneda at 10:00 A.M. and at 1:30 P.M. climbed aboard a C-54 military aircraft bound for Sapporo. They arrived at Chitose airbase, which is located about 30 miles east of Sapporo, and traveled to the Grand Hotel by car, arriving about 6:45 P.M. Colonel Hall, the chief liaison officer for Camp Crawford and commanding officer of the 13th Station hospital, visited the hotel to have dinner with Drs. Seevers and Darrow. On Sunday evening, Dr. Yashuda, dean of Hokkaido University School of Medicine, paid a courtesy call to Dr. Seevers. They met at the station hospital as guests of Colonel Hall.

At 10:00 A.M. on Monday, the mission members were given an official welcome by Vice-Governor Fukuda, president of Hokkaido University, along with the deans of two medical schools in Sapporo. In the afternoon, Dr. Seevers met faculty members Dr. Masaki and myself, to make plans for the two-week stay. At 4:00 P.M., the president of Hokkaido University had a tea reception which included beer and a buffet-style banquet. Dr. Seevers said that the Sapporo beer was the best in Japan and the best beer he had ever tasted. Furthermore, it lacked the hangover effect of American beer! The governor of Hokkaido arranged a special presentation of a fabulous puppet show which was performed by the number one puppeteer in Japan who happened to be visiting from Osaka. After the performance, the mission members were taken backstage to meet the manipulators and had a chance to operate the puppets themselves.

Dr. Seevers gave lectures to the students and held staff conferences at Hokkaido University School of Medicine and Sapporo Medical College during the mornings almost every day. My staff took notes at his lectures and prepared a notebook for their own purpose. Dr. Masaki, the chairman of the Department of Pharmacology, added a preface to the

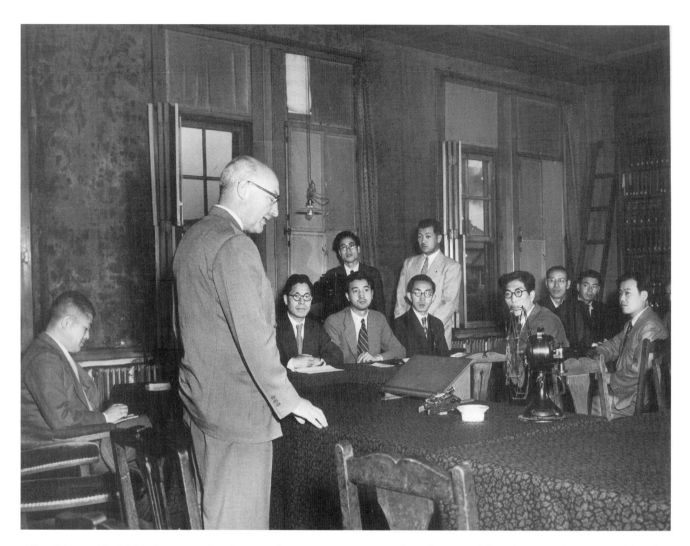

Fig. 4. June 12, 1951, Sapporo. Dr. Seevers lectures to a group of students and faculty members at Hokkaido University Medical School. Behind Dr. Seevers is Dr. Hosoya and immediately to his right Dr. Tanabe.

notebook. The table of contents of the notes is as follows:

A. Lectures for the students

B. Staff Conferences

In his lectures, Dr. Seevers referred to important achievements by American pharmacologists in recent years. The lectures were clearly translated into Japanese by Dr. Hosoya. The notes were corrected by both interpreters, Drs. Kumagai and Hosoya, and were hand copied as a memento of their attendance.

Dr. Seevers was also busy with invitations to luncheons and dinners from many influential persons in Sapporo; he became a welcomed guest because of his open-hearted and frank yet gentlemanly ways. I think that Dr. Seevers also felt very happy with the good mutual relationship and inter-reliance be-

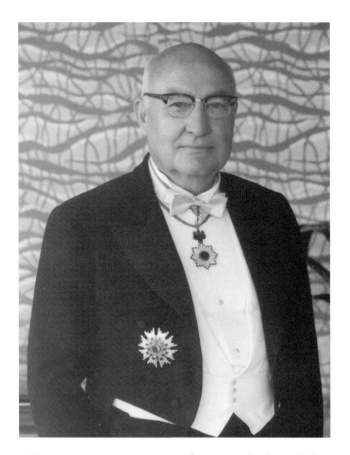

Fig. 5. Dr. Seevers wearing the Second Class of the Order of the Sacred Treasure (breast) and The Third Class of the Order of the Rising Sun Medal (neck) given by the Japanese government in Tokyo in 1967.

tween fellow scientists of the two different countries. Subsequently, he raised funds for young Japanese pharmacologists to study in his laboratory in Ann Arbor. He also visited Japan very often afterwards to maintain communication with fellow Japanese pharmacologists.

The educational funds raised by Dr. Seevers consisted of two types, one for study tours of short duration for senior pharmacologists, and the other for junior pharmacologists of one or more years. Through his interest and generosity, the level of competency of Japanese pharmacology has been raised at the University of Michigan. The Japanese government recognized Dr. Seevers' distinguished service and decorated him with the Second Order of the Sacred Treasure of Japan.

The Beginnings of Japanese Seevers Michigan Fellows: 1952 and Beyond

Eikichi Hosoya, M.D., Ph.D.

The intimate relationship between the University of Michigan Department of Pharmacology and Japanese pharmacology originated from the Second U.S. Medical Mission sponsored by the Unitarian Service (a religious foundation in the United States) and the U.S. Department of the Army. Brig. General Dr. Crawford F. Sams of the General Headquarters of the U.S. Occupation Forces strongly requested that the advances of U.S. medicine be made available in Japan. He held the responsibility for the health and welfare of the Japanese people at the time of the Occupation.

In 1950, the first medical mission visited Japan. The aim of the mission was to elevate the level of knowledge among Japanese medical scientists. All the professors in Japanese medical schools were requested to attend the lecture course Monday through Friday for two weeks in Tokyo, Kobe, or Sapporo. Although many professors, at first, felt uncomfortable in being given such orders, their eyes were quickly opened and they recognized the rapid advances in basic and clinical medicine made in the U.S. during World War II. Accordingly, many participants were inclined to hear and learn from the lectures, which were a success. In the field of pharmacology, Dr. McKeen Cattell of Cornell University lectured on the pharmacology of drugs for heart diseases. These were splendid lectures originating from his life-long research.

Following the success of the first, a second medical mission (head: Paul Beeson, M.D.; secretary, Miss Snavely) was sent to Japan in May of the next year, 1951. Dr. Maurice Harrison Seevers of the University of Michigan was a member of this second mission. He talked mainly on central nervous system (CNS) pharmacology including drug dependence. These lectures were held in the same cities as the first series, but the participants were not limited to professors; also included were the medical school students. The latter received an even stronger impact from the lectures than the older professors and were more receptive to recognizing the high level of the U.S. medical sciences, pharmacology in particular.

Fortunately, I attended both rounds of courses and was asked to be the interpreter for Dr. Seevers' lectures in Tokyo and Sapporo. I was not good at speaking English, and interpretation needs understanding and expression simultaneously. Because of this, I hesitated to accept the job, but the recommendation of Dr. Cattell and the kind invitation of Dr. Seevers led me to accept. Dr. Seevers' lectures to the audiences were easy to understand and his explanations were not difficult to interpret. Thinking back on the lectures, I don't believe I made many mistakes. The number of attendees was around 150. I do not know how many schools of medicine and pharmaceutical science existed at that time in

Japan, so the exact number of attendees is not clear. I believe that one to three pharmacologists from each medical school attended Seevers' lectures. M.H. Seevers gradually came to be know among Japanese pharmacologists as "the specialist on CNS drugs."

The biggest pleasure for me was the kind and thoughtful attitude of Dr. Seevers toward the Japanese, not only in the lecture hall, but also in the hotels and restaurants after the lectures. I accompanied him all day and found my mind relaxed by his joyous nature. Thus, it was quite natural that I chose the Department of Pharmacology at the University of Michigan when I was nominated as a Fellow of the Rockefeller Foundation (1952–53). Moreover, after that one year, Dr. Seevers appointed me as an instructor in his department.

I have heard many favorable stories of many different U.S. professors taking very good care of Japanese fellows. I believe the mutual respect and affection I share with the Seevers family may be one of the best. My wife, Kimi, respected and loved Mrs. Frances (Frankie) Seevers with all her heart. My son, Hideo, studied in the same class with Dr. Seevers' son Giles under Mrs. Newcomb at Angell Elementary School in Ann Arbor, Michigan. Giles sometimes asked my wife for a little pocket money. Similarly, my son would open the freezer in the Seevers' kitchen without permission to get some ice cream. The children played happily and quarreled, too, in and out of the classroom. My wife and I were surprised how fast my son learned many bad names to call others. So, the Seevers and the Hosoyas came to act more like relatives than just neighbors. My wife and I were introduced to all of the intimate friends of the Seevers, such as the Sheldons and the Nesbits, with whom we associated as naturally as old friends.

The morning of my first visit to the Department of Pharmacology at Michigan, Dr. Lauren Woods took me to the pharmacology building. It was an old three story building on the left side of the Diag directly opposite the University Library. It was in Ann Arbor that the first lecture on pharmacology had been given by Dr. John Jacob Abel in 1891.

Lauren Woods was a typical American gentleman. I don't remember how many times we were invited to his home located in a woods in Barton Hills. I used to joke, "the Woods live in the woods." My son liked to play in the woods with the children of Lauren's family like Tarzan in the movies. I had heard that Lauren Woods was a graduate of the University of Michigan Medical School with a straight A record in all of his courses. The Woods family were refined, intelligent, tender, thoughtful, and religious, and not at all self-serving. I sometimes thought that if Dr. Woods had been a self-promoting pharmacologist, he would have risen to a very high money-earning position in the world of medical science. As it turned out, he achieved a very enviable stature because of his contributions to pharmacology, chemistry, and medical education. For many years, I visited the Woods in Iowa and in Virginia where they went after leaving Michigan. They enjoyed peaceful and productive lives.

When I first arrived in Ann Arbor, I told Dr. Seevers that I did not need a degree but was anxious to learn the latest advancements in CNS pharmacology. He recommended that I study with Dr. Theodore Brody, who had worked previously with Dr. Bain. Ted was a recipient of the Abel Award for a unique theory on anesthesia. Ted had come to Ann Arbor a few weeks before I had, in 1952. As Ted had no assistant, I worked very hard under his direction, chiefly on the changes of phosphorus to oxygen ratio by various compounds using cat or rat papillary muscles. Ted taught me in detail his latest research methods. I feel many obligations to him even now. At the same time, I should add that this was the hardest period of my research life. After one year's hard work with Ted, the direction of my study turned to the metabolism of morphine in the living body. This was an important subject about which I had first learned

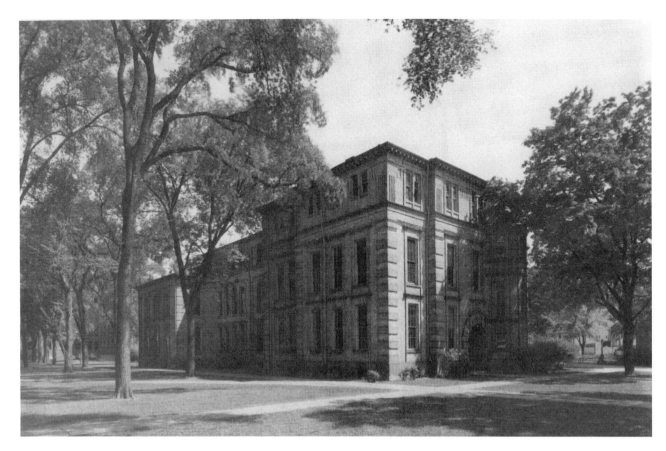

Fig. 1. The Pharmacology Building on the Diag. Home of Materia Medica/Pharmacology, 1910–1958. Originally the Chemistry Building, the first portion of this structure was built in 1856. After numerous additions and improvements, it was assigned to Physiology and Materia Medica in 1910. In the 1920s, Physiology moved to the new East Medical Building. The Department of Pharmacology moved from this structure to Medical Science Building I in 1958. In its last years, part of the old building housed the Department of Economics. On Christmas Eve, 1981, it was set afire by an arsonist and was subsequently razed.

from Dr. K. Abe at Keio University. Together with several assistants, I worked mainly on the conjugation of morphine with glucuronic acid.

Beyond the Woods and the Brodys, we associated with almost all members of the department. Because of their thoughtfulness, my family and I never felt inferior throughout our two-year stay in Ann Arbor.

The more I think back, the more reminiscences come to mind. Many people say that the 1950s was the best decade in the history of the U.S.; I would agree. For example, my son left his overcoat on a bench in a park one afternoon and the next morning I found it as it had been left, without anything lost or stolen. Though small in population, Ann Arbor was

really an academic city consisting chiefly of intellectual people. We heard of no robbery, killing, or violence in Ann Arbor at that time. This was in contrast to Detroit or Chicago where all kinds of crimes occurred continuously.

In the spring, a May festival was held in Hill Auditorium. In the fall, the young and old sang the alma mater together in Michigan's huge football stadium. My wife enjoyed shopping at Jacobson's with Frankie Seevers. I often bought bottles of apple cider at the Farmer's Market. After one and a half years in Ann Arbor, my wife and I discussed seriously whether we should apply for U.S. citizenship to stay longer in the U.S. However, we came to the conclusion that although we were en-

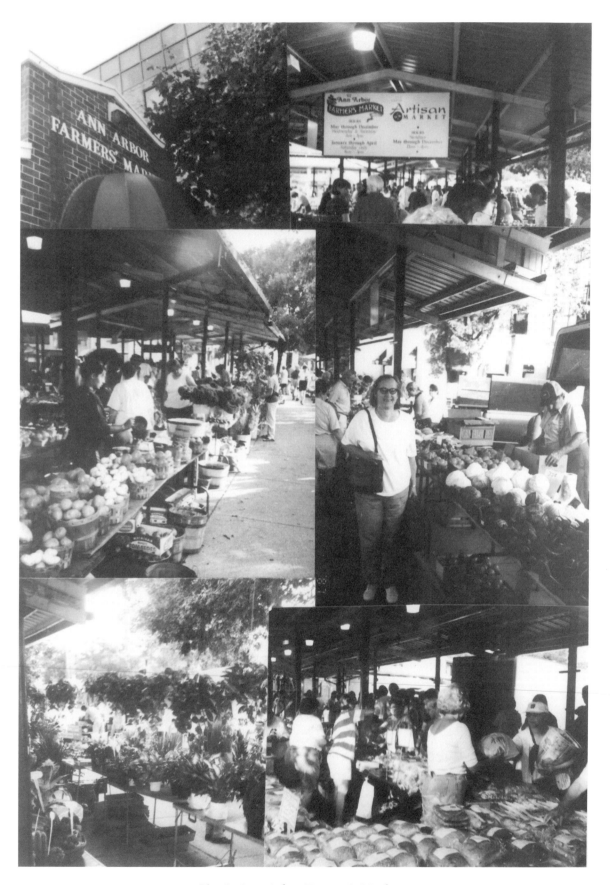

Fig. 2. Ann Arbor Farmer's Market.

joying a happy life there, it was because we were guests in the U.S. With my abilities, I would not be able to attain the rank of professor in a U.S. medical school. So, my wife and I gave up our idea to apply for U.S. citizenship. When the time came for us to leave Ann Arbor after a full two years' stay, we stopped at the Seevers' house to say farewell; we could not keep from crying. I noticed dew in the eyes of Dr. Seevers and Frankie also.

A few days before my departure, Dr. Seevers clearly told me "You have done well. I am sorry to lose you but I have been able to find a good sponsor who is willing to pay the expenses of Japanese pharmacologists who would like to study in our department for a year. Please look for one or two able young Japanese researchers annually and send me their names and curriculum vitae. I will write a letter of invitation to whomever you think best. I leave the decision on who to select exclusively to you." These words of Dr. Seevers led to the start of the Michigan fellowships from Japan. He kept his promise firmly until his retirement. Since I knew that Dr. Seevers got along well with Dr. Tanabe from Sapporo, I suggested his name during the first discussion on Michigan fellows; Dr. Seevers agreed instantly. Thus, the first Michigan fellow from Japan was decided very quickly. However, finding the best Japanese candidates for University of Michigan pharmacology remained a big concern for me over a period of 20 years.

In 1956, Dr. Seevers visited Japan for the second time as the head of a medical mission on anesthesiology. As before, I accompanied him on his travels through Japan. The lectures on anesthesiology were held in Tokyo, Kyoto, Fukuoka, and Sapporo. I cannot recall the names of the lecturers in full, but the names of Drs. Wescoe, Riker, Shideman, and Artusio come to mind. During our stay in Kyoto, I thought Dr. Hiroshi Takagi from Kyoto University would be a good candidate as a Michigan fellow and asked Dr. Seevers his opinion. Dr. Seevers agreed with me and I asked Dr. Takagi whether or not he could go to Ann Arbor. Surprisingly, his answer was no be-

cause one day earlier he had promised Dr. Riker that he would go to Cornell University. Dr. Seevers and I felt very sorry that we were too late in this case. Looking back on Dr. Takagi's work at Cornell, he succeeded splendidly in studies on analgesic mechanisms in living animals. I think even now, as far as analgesics are concerned, I wish he had studied at the University of Michigan rather than at Cornell.

After Kyoto, we went to Fukuoka where we would find a good substitute for Dr. Takagi. Dr. Ueki, assistant professor in the Department of Pharmacology at Kyushu University, was an able man with a vast knowledge of the central nervous system. Though small in physical stature, he was a giant in research enthusiasm. He instantly accepted our invitation with pleasure. After a year, I met Dr. Ueki in Ann Arbor and heard from him that he was studying happily with Dr. Edward F. Domino. After he became professor of pharmacology at the Pharmaceutical School of Kyushu University, his abilities blossomed widely and powerfully. In a few years, he became a major influence in the southwestern area of the Japanese Pharmacological Society. Later, he was nominated for presidency of the Japanese Pharmaceutical Society. His main interest was in clinical pharmacology even though he was not teaching in a medical school. His students are now scattered throughout the southwestern area of Japan as professors of pharmacology in medical and pharmaceutical chemistry schools, as well as in the pharmaceutical industry.

After the first and second experiences in the selection of Michigan fellows, I made some general rules concerning the selection of candidates as follows:

1. The aim of Dr. Seevers is to elevate the level of Japanese pharmacology. Therefore, only superior candidates must be selected.
2. The candidates must come from all over Japan, not only from first class universities in big cities.

3. The candidates may be interested in any aspect of the wide field of pharmacology.

4. Preferred candidates are to be assistant professors or instructors in Japanese medical or pharmaceutical chemistry schools who are willing to spend their future in pharmacological research, not necessarily in pharmaceutical industry.

5. Applications or recommendations of candidates will be accepted all year round, but at least one year in advance.

6. Applicants must not only be capable in the pharmacological sciences, but also show a spirit of cooperation with the members of Seevers' department. Proficiency in English conversation is not absolutely necessary but, for some, extra education at the English Language Institute in Ann Arbor may be required.

7. When a suitable candidate is found, a personal interview is indispensable as the circumstances and will of the applicant must be confirmed.

8. No group, especially any academic organization, may be completely neglected.

9. The Japanese Pharmacological Society consists of four geographically divided parts.

   a) North (includes Niigata, Sendai, Sapporo)
   b) Kanto (Tokyo and its suburbs)
   c) Kinki (Kyoto, Osaka, Nagoya, Hiroshima)
   d) Southwest (Kyushu, Shikoku, Okinawa)

   When there is only one candidate, he will be selected either from the (a+b) parts or (c+d) parts alternately. If two candidates can be accepted, one should be selected from the (a+b) parts and one from the (c+d) parts. This way the distribution of Michigan fellows will cover all of Japan. (Looking back, this aim was very suitable.)

10. According to the above rules, a candidate is to be roughly screened, then I will request the opinion of Drs. Kumagai and Yamada, professors of pharmacology at the Universities of Tokyo and Kyoto, respectively. (No opposition ever came from either of them.)

11. Finally, all the information on the candidates will be sent to Dr. Seevers. (Dr. Seevers wrote to me in 1976 as follows: "The selection of Michigan fellows gives me great satisfaction that all of these fellows have returned to Japan and occupy positions of major responsibility in Japanese Pharmacology.")

Of course, there arose a few contradictions or doubts in practicing the above rules accurately. There were several cases in which I was in doubt between two candidates, as in the case of Drs. Murayama and Yanagita. Finally, Dr. Nakao, the teacher of Yanagita,

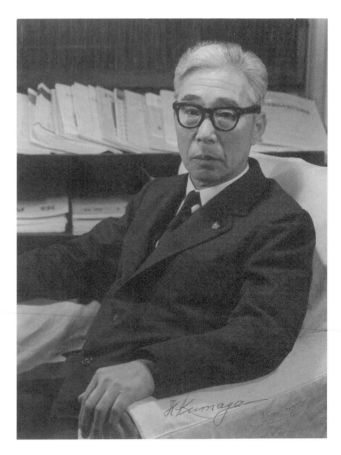

Fig. 3. Dr. Hiroshi Kumagai, Professor and Chairman, Department of Pharmacology, Tokyo University Faculty of Medicine established a close tie between UM Pharmacology and the Japanese Pharmacological Society through Dr. M.H. Seevers.

stated that their medical school, Jikei, was a private school and got relatively few grants compared to national universities such as Chiba (Murayama's school). Dr. Nakao emphasized this issue and asked me to be in favor of Yanagita. I agreed to recommend him to Dr. Seevers, but I was greatly concerned about Dr. Murayama and his loss of opportunity. Happily, in less than a year Dr. Murayama found other support to go to the University of Illinois. In later years, Dr. Murayama was elected president of the Japanese Pharmacological Society, while Dr. Yanagita established a unique method to evaluate the psychic dependence in monkeys under the guidance of Dr. Seevers. Readers may realize how difficult it is to discriminate between two outstanding candidates with equal levels of ability.

The case of Dr. Yamamoto, who was working at the Shionogi Research Institute which belonged to the Shionogi Pharmaceutical Company, involved the first part of rule four. Dr. Tokizane, professor of physiology at the University of Tokyo, insisted that the development of Dr. Yamamoto's career under the direction of Dr. Edward Domino would undoubtedly encourage the development of pharmacological EEG studies in Japan. I finally accepted his recommendation to strengthen relationships with the pharmaceutical industry in Japan.

Not only the Seevers Michigan Fellows but also other Japanese pharmacologists went to Ann Arbor for further training. The names of all of the fellows from Japan who went to the Department of Pharmacology at Michigan are so numerous that I am unable to list them. The thick book *U.S. and Japan* published by Asahi Newspaper Company stated, "Ann Arbor is a mecca for Japanese pharmacologists now." I have always felt sincere gratitude and a little pride that I was involved.

As the number of Michigan fellows increased, unanticipated powers have been felt in the Japanese Pharmacological Society. Since every fellow has been very active and able, their society influences in Japan are obvious. It was not the purpose of Dr. Seevers to create a special clique, but rather to raise the level of all Japanese pharmacology. The Michigan fellows did not run for election as president, councilors, or other positions in the Japanese Pharmacological Society simply for self-promotion. It was good that each individual fellow continuously published excellent scientific results, which propelled each of them into appropriate high positions. That is one of the reasons why the Michigan fellows group could continue for so long without creating jealousy or conflict.

There are 48 medical schools in Japan, each with one or two professors of pharmacology. Almost all Michigan fellows have become professors of pharmacology in medical or pharmaceutical science schools. If Dr. Seevers were alive today, he would be glad that his dream came true and that the activities of the Japanese Pharmacological Society, especially of the Seevers Michigan Fellows, have flourished.

It is my duty to describe the hidden financial and moral support of Dr. Walter A. Compton for the Seevers Michigan Fellows. If a man wishes to write on Michigan fellows, the name of Dr. Walter Compton must never be neglected. Dr. Compton was well known as the former president of Miles Laboratory Inc. in Elkhart, Indiana. He was an intimate friend of Dr. Seevers. He had degrees in chemistry (Princeton University) and medicine (Harvard) and was a most intelligent scientist and businessman. Many of the expenses of the Michigan fellows were paid by Dr. Compton, a fact which he did not want to be known. It was forbidden even to speak about his support for a long time, although the reason was never revealed. . After several of Dr. Seevers' visits to Japan, Dr. Compton accompanied him. All of the Michigan fellows treated Dr. Seevers as nicely as possible. However, Dr. Compton was not treated as nicely as Dr. Seevers since he was considered an outsider. Dr. Seevers requested the same treatment be given to Dr. Compton as to himself.

Dr. Compton was very pro-Japanese. He

returned to the Japanese government a sword (engraved Kunimune) which had been a national treasure of Japan before the war, and also famous pictures drawn by Miyamoto Musashi (the most famous swordsman in Japanese history as well as a painter) without receiving any reward. He did appropriately receive a medal of honor for his gifts to Japan. I visited him in Elkhart, Indiana three times and stayed at his home twice. He lived in a big house with a large underground room which was used for his collection of world famous items such as a violin by Stradivarius and many Japanese swords, tsuba and inroh (medicine cases). I was surprised by his gorgeous collection and its inestimable value. He especially loved Japanese swords (katana), kept carefully from extremes of humidity, temperature, and dust. He could read the engraving of the name of the sword maker in Japanese and always tested my knowledge of Japanese sword makers.

It is also appropriate to refer to another hidden supporter of the Seevers Michigan Fellows in Japan. Tsusai Sugawara was an unusual and powerful politician (the unrealized "Mayor of Tokyo"). He was the strongest leader of the Antinarcotic Association of Japan (a non-governmental organization for the banishment of three national evils: narcotics, prostitution, and venereal disease). He protested against narcotics every day and everywhere. Having known the name of Dr. Seevers since he and I were councilors of the Japanese cabinet on narcotics, he invited Dr. Seevers to his home in Kamakura, a huge old house filled with many antique objects. He spoke enthusiastically about his activities against narcotics and asked for scientific help from Dr. Seevers. Dr. Seevers, of course, agreed and promised to make speeches whenever necessary. Their relationship became very close. Two medals of honor from the Japanese government which Dr. Seevers received were the result of the efforts of Mr. Sugawara and myself. I will never forget the happy face of Dr. Seevers when the medals (Sacred Treasure 2nd Class and Rising

Sun 3rd Class) were pinned on his chest by the Minister of the Government. Dr. Seevers called Mr. Sugawara "a magnificent man" and asked the president of the University of Michigan to invite him to the president's guest house in Ann Arbor; this was done. The contribution of Mr. Sugawara to the Department of Pharmacology at the University of Michigan was spiritual and political, rather than financial, but just as important.

Dr. Seevers had a special interest in Japanese bonsai. We both became members of the Japan Bonsai Society. Not only did he visit many exhibitions of bonsai around Tokyo, he also went to Shikoku to inspect the big collection of Ishizuchi-goyo-matsu (pine trees with five leaves, chiefly growing on the Ishizuchi mountain, in Shikoku) which a friend of mine kept in his garden. He admired the techniques by which Japanese people bred natural trees to such a small size, caring for them for several hundred years and through many generations. He purchased bonsai several times and tried to take them back home. Alas, because U.S. customs were very strict about the importation of foreign plants, the soil was completely brushed out and disinfectant poured on the roots. None of the bonsai brought back could survive. Dr. Seevers had a medium-sized greenhouse in his basement where he tried to breed bonsai, but despite his enthusiasm his attempts were not satisfactory. He even drove to Rocky Mountain National Park to pick up bonsai-styled trees, but they were too big to be true bonsai. Eventually, Dr. Seevers was able to collect and grow many bonsai in his greenhouse and in the summer outdoors.

After he passed away, most were given to the University of Michigan Matthaei Botanical Gardens (see Appendix C). I think Dr. Seevers was a rare American who understood elegant Japanese manners and customs. This was symbolized by his request for a yukimotoro (a snow-viewing lantern, with a large top and tripod, all made of stone).

Dr. Seevers was kind enough to intro-

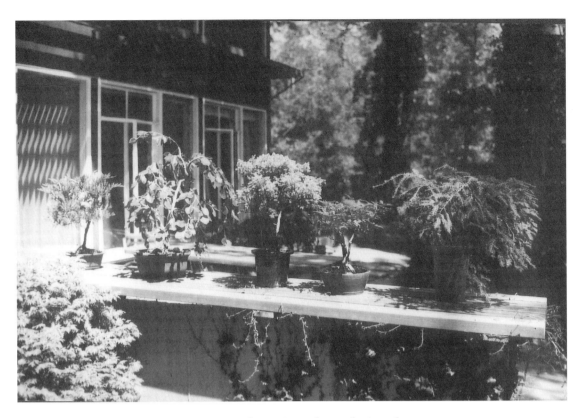

Fig. 4. Some Seevers' bonsai outdoors during the summer.

duce me to many scholars, not only pharmacologists in the U.S. but also other world-famous medical scientists at every occasion. I attended the Congress of the International Union of Pharmacology (IUPHAR) from its first meeting in Stockholm until the 11th meeting in Mannheim, and came to know many eminent specialists worldwide. That may be the reason why I was nominated as a member of the International Advisory Board of IUPHAR (1971, Palo Alto). I served as co-chairman of the all-day symposium on drugs and society, co-chaired by Dr. E.L. Way, at the congress held in San Francisco in 1972. Moreover, in the general assembly, I was elected a councilor of IUPHAR, which I owed to the efforts of Drs. Seevers and Bain. At the general assembly of IUPHAR in Helsinki in 1975, I was nominated as second vice-president of IUPHAR. It was the first time the position had been offered to an Asian pharmacologist.

In Japan, I was a councilor of the Japanese Pharmacological Society for a long time until my retirement from Keio University Medical School. I was elected president of the Japanese Pharmacological Society in 1970. Five years earlier, I had also been nominated as a member of the WHO Expert Panel on Drug Abuse, a position which I held for 12 years.

I traveled outside of Japan 77 times until the age of 80, including 30 times to the U.S., 20 times to Europe, seven times to China, and three times each to Russia and Australia. It was a big pleasure when I could meet other pharmacologists who were studying in Ann Arbor, such as Dr. Pardo (Mexico), Dr. Mukerji (India), Dr. Pensritong (Thailand), and Dr. Kaymakçalan (Turkey). In 1958, I succeeded in establishing a cooperative group to study drug abuse between the National Science Foundation (U.S.) and the Japan Society for the Promotion of Science. The chairman in the U.S. was Dr. N.B. Eddy and the co-chairman was Dr. Seevers. On the Japanese side, I was chairman and Dr. Kasamatsu (professor of psychiatry at the University of Tokyo) was co-chairman. Our mutual cooperation continued for six years. The funds from the two governments were insufficient, but each member spent some useful time in the U.S. and Japan. Dr. Eddy wrote a record of the activity of this group in his books *Status of the U.S.-Japan Cooperative Science Program, March 31, 1967* and *The National Research Council Involvement in the Opiate Problem 1928–1971.*

After my retirement from Keio University Medical School, the General Congress of IUPHAR was held in Tokyo (president, Dr. Ebashi). I invited some of my old pharmacology acquaintances from around the world. The guests numbered 60, and there were only two absentees, Dr. E.L. Way and Dr. Hollister. After retirement, I turned my interests around 180 degrees to study traditional Chinese medicine using modern methodology. I was appointed first to the Kanebo Pharmaceutical Company in 1974, and four years later moved to the Tsumura Company, chiefly managing research and development of traditional Chinese medicine.

I served on the editorial boards of the *Japanese Journal of Pharmacology* and *Folia Pharmacologica Japonica* for at least 10 years as a member of the advisory board of *Pharmacological Communications* (Academic Press). *Trends in Pharmacological Science* (*TIPS*) was published when I was vice-president of IUPHAR. Inasmuch as Dr. Burns, the president, had big expectations for *TIPS*, I agreed to participate as a member of the editorial board in order to accelerate contributions from Japan. I retired from the board in 1992 after 13 years of service.

If my memory is correct, Dr. Seevers came to Japan 23 times and I accompanied him every time. I can honestly say that he loved Japan and the Japanese people. After the death of Dr. Seevers, my affection for his wife, Frankie, and vice versa, continued unaltered. Because of my advancing age, my concern with the Department of Pharmacology at the University of Michigan decreased gradually. Communications between Japan and

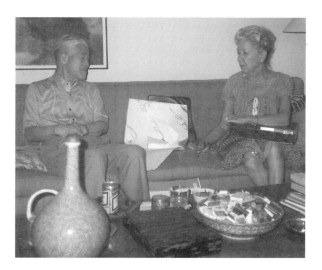

Fig. 5. Dr. Hosoya visiting Frankie Seevers in Ann Arbor, 1983.

Ann Arbor were chiefly handled by Dr. Yanagita. I made little contribution to more recent Michigan fellowships. As time passes, such events are handled by the younger generation of Japanese pharmacologists.

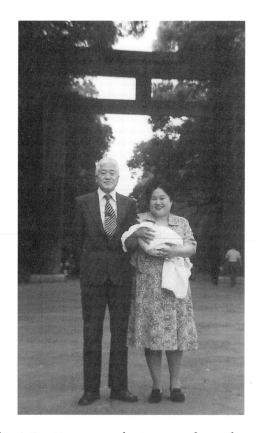

Fig. 6. Dr. Hosoya, wife, Kimi, and grandson in Tokyo.

5

Excerpts from the Diary Letters of
Dr. Maurice H. Seevers on His First Visit to Japan

◄○►

Maurice H. Seevers, M.D., Ph.D.

Sunday, 13 May 1951,
Dai-Ichi Hotel, Tokyo

It all seems like a dream. This hotel is a fabulous place, the atmosphere of which is difficult to describe by American comparisons. It was built in preparation for the Olympic Games which never materialized here. It is the second best hotel in Tokyo; the Imperial is number one. We will be here for about two weeks. Our whole group moves south after Tokyo and then north. I go to the northernmost island of Hokkaido which contains a few of the original occupants of Japan. We will have a conference this morning with Dr. Kusama, president of the Japanese Medical Society, and tomorrow begins the rounds. . . .

Monday, 14 May 1951, Dai-Ichi Hotel

I just crawled out of the bathtub. It is a dandy. I cannot sit with my knees completely straight and need a can opener to get out. The electrical railroad runs down the street in front of the hotel and makes a considerable racket with the peculiar beep-beep of its whistle. During the quiet of the night, one can hear the occasional train roll by, and in the intervening periods the clatter of the *geta,* the wooden shoes worn by the poorer and older people. The shoes clack-clack along the street and the sound reverberates in the still air.

Yesterday morning we spent some time with Dr. Kusama, a Stanford-trained man, one of the few American graduates in Japan. He has been encouraged by the Supreme Commander of the Allied Powers (SCAP) because of his knowledge of English and American methods. Whether he will be able to hold his position after the Treaty of Peace is signed is doubtful since he is at Keio University and traditionally Tokyo University is more important. Dr. Kusama told us about medical education in Japan. There were 76 medical schools during the war, many very poor. This is now reduced to 46 medical schools of two classes, some often accepting students with merely a high school education. We will go only to the best. After this discussion, we went to the headquarters of Public Health and Welfare (PH&W) to look at all the drugs which I had obtained from U.S. industry. They are probably worth between $5,000 and $10,000. They will be well received, I am sure.

We will go to Tokyo University to meet the faculty and arrange for our program. Evidently we are going to be permitted to lecture to the Japanese students. . . .

Tuesday, 15 May 1951, Dai-Ichi Hotel

I haven't yet got adjusted to hearing the clatter of the *geta* and the elevated train. Furthermore, there just isn't any time to get writing done with the push of things. I have had to reorganize all my slides and lectures since I didn't get much chance before we left. The desire to see this fabulous place keeps us meandering around the streets in the evenings. Tokyo never sleeps. The shops seem to be open all of the time, day or night, seven days a week.

Monday morning we had a briefing by General Sams, who is in charge of the PH&W section. He has done a remarkable job in public health over a period of five years. As an example, 80,000 Japanese have been vaccinated for smallpox. Only five cases were found in Japan in 1950. The death rate from TB and intestinal dysenteries, etc. has been greatly reduced. Life expectancy in the males has been increased from 43 to 56 years during this period.

At 10:30 A.M. we went to Tokyo University for our first Japanese contact. Dr. Lucia (preventive medicine, U. Of Columbia), Dr. Darrow (pediatrics, Yale) and I are on the team at Tokyo University. We met Dean Kodama, my counterpart in pharmacology, Professor Kobayashi, and the other professors in this group. We arranged our program for the two-week period. This activity took until noon and after lunch at the Dai-Ichi we continued into the afternoon. I was then introduced to the Department of Pharmacology by Dr. Kobayashi and my interpreter, Dr. Hosoya, assistant professor of pharmacology at Keio University here in Tokyo. He is a fine lad. All of the professors of pharmacology in the Tokyo area and their assistants were waiting. I was introduced to the group and we had tea. This was only an introductory affair and I was ceremoniously given a key to a nice office to use during my stay in Tokyo. The Japanese are very gracious people indeed.

We had to leave early today in order to make an engagement with the Minister of Education of Japan who threw a party for us in a beautiful restaurant in Ueno Park. It was attended by the presidents and deans, many professors emeriti, and by dignitaries in the ministry and military. After the introductions, we were conducted to a large room with tables at which we sat in groups of six or eight at each table. On each table were dishes of peanuts, sliced cheese and crackers. A buffet

dinner was served along with Japanese beer which is more like our ale and equally as potent. Glasses were never permitted to become empty. After an introductory speech by Minister Odono, its interpretation, a reply by our chairman (Dr. Beeson of Emory) and its translation, we enjoyed a meal.

During the evening meal, we were entertained by two girls playing the Koto, a 13-stringed instrument about six feet long having movable bridges, one under each string, which the player moves with the left hand as she plays in order to get the proper tones. It is an amazing instrument and requires extensive training of the ear to recognize tone differences. It probably corresponds as closely to our piano as anything, but is infinitely more difficult to play. Two beautiful Japanese girls, one an instructor in the leading Japanese dancing school, entertained us. Their dancing and costumes were really beautiful and their grace and delicate interpretation was something not seen in other types of dance. Perry Volpitto took pictures during the performance and after the affair was over the performers were introduced to everyone. Pictures were taken of the group and the entertainers collectively and individually to the great merriment of all, especially the older Japanese. It was a gala occasion and probably as good an example of the Japanese dance as we will see or, in fact, is available. . . .

Wednesday, 16 May 1951, Dai-Ichi Hotel

Tuesday morning I spent at the Kakubu Building SCAP headquarters of PH&W, dividing the drugs into 12 lots for distribution to medical schools which we intend to visit. We then loaded them in a jeep and took them to the hotel and had lunch, then Dr. Darrow and I took off for Tokyo University about 1:30 P.M. We arrived there about 2:45 P.M. and I went to the pharmacology department where we unloaded the stuff to the great excitement of the assistants and even the professor. The other professors were all assembled. The drug allotments were made to Tokyo, Keio, Jikei-Kai and Chiba Universities. I then began my first staff conference with Japanese men from eight to 10 universities and their assistants. I talked on "Newer Synthetic Analgesics." This group understood English well enough to permit the interpreter to only summarize my talk about every 10 minutes. Slides help a great deal. They all seemed to be very interested and asked numerous questions. As a special honor, Professor Kobayashi presented me with a letter expressing his gratitude. When we finished up at about 4:00 P.M. we couldn't find our Army driver. We were driven to the Dai-Ichi by the chauffeur of the president of Tokyo University (a real imposition since the Japanese are rationed on gasoline and really cannot afford it).

This country is poverty stricken and the populace scrimp and save everything. They are very gracious, however, about spending money. The salary of my interpreter, Dr. Hosoya, is 14,000 yen per month which is $40. This chap has two children. His wife is also a physician and helps support them by working in a maternal health clinic. . . .

Thursday, 17 May 1951, Dai-Ichi Hotel
Yesterday was a big thrill. I do not believe an American has ever lectured to a group of students of medicine in Japan on pharmacology before today. It was a real experience. We went to the University about 9:00 A.M. and I spent the first hour discussing the lectures with my interpreter, Dr. Hosoya. Dr. Kobayashi came in about 9:45 and showed me a copy of his speech to the Japanese students. I was then conducted ceremoniously into the amphitheater which is much better than any we have at Michigan. The class of 130 students had assembled as well as a large number of others from the faculty and surrounding environs. I was instructed to talk slowly so that the students would understand. I honestly believe they did get most of it, although it is difficult to determine exactly. My interpreter summarized about every five minutes. I talked again on "Morphine and the Newer

Synthetics." I only saw one kid sleeping during the whole period, which is an accomplishment. I guess they were interested in the whole phenomenon.

We returned to Tokyo for a conference with Professor Kobayashi and his staff. He wanted to discuss our respective departments so we exchanged information. The Japanese are very anxious to talk about their research and they must be given the opportunity. Drs. Kumagai, Uraguchi and Hosoya were present. After the discussion, Dr. Hosoya wanted to take us to a Japanese restaurant for dinner but we begged off and went to a Shinto shrine instead. The Meiji Shrine is one of the three largest in Japan, located in the center of a beautiful park. This shrine was virtually laid waste by fire in the bombing of Tokyo. In fact, nearly everything of real value was mostly destroyed except those things made of brick and stone. However, the Japanese do not seem to be too greatly perturbed about losing their homes. Every Japanese expects to lose everything he has about three times in his lifetime, either from earthquake, typhoon, or fire.

The Japanese children are really cute and there are plenty of them of all ages on the streets. Boys and girls about 10-12 years old go on hikes with their knapsacks on their backs, sometimes several hundred in one group. I saw a string of them yesterday which stretched out for over a block. We also saw a Shinto ceremonial parade of about 30–40 little kids, ages four to seven, pulling and riding a large float on wheels which had a paper egg on it as large as our kitchen stove. All of the kids had on kimonos of beautiful colors and there were many colored ribbons running to the float. Some of the older kids wore a harness which was attached for pulling the float. It was a very colorful affair.

PH&W is in a stew. It appears as if it will be closed up soon and possibly the Peace Treaty will be signed by July 1. We must be home by then since no money is available for payment of per diem after that. . . .

Friday, 18 May 1951, Dai-Ichi Hotel

The mad pace continues. We don't seem to have more than a minute to sit down. We could be engaged in 10 more activities but physical endurance will not permit it. Yesterday, our team spent the morning in the clinical field. We listened to an excellent lecture and demonstration of a patient by Professor Wakemoto. Although we had an interpreter, it was clear that Professor Wakemoto was an excellent teacher. The students were permitted to cursorily examine the patient. They do not usually touch a patient, but defer to the assistance of a professor; there may be as many as a hundred students. Ward rounds simulate a parade. The medical clinic was held in a large amphitheater which must be 40 feet tall. It had fine paneled wood and two sets of galleries. The young men at the top could barely see the proceedings (as is the case in some U.S. clinics).

After visiting the clinic, we visited the hospital wards. All Japanese hospitals are the same; the family moves in and takes care of the patient except for medications. There is a central dietary kitchen that is supposed to supply the hospital, but there seems to be as much cooking going on in the wards as ever. The operating rooms are kept wet and one wears wooden *geta* or slipovers upon entering. We saw a surgical amphitheater where two or three patients were being operated on at the same time. No one but the surgeon wears gloves and there are many hands in the incision. A nurse takes the bloody sponges from the wound, carefully washes them, and puts them back on the stand. Anesthesia just doesn't exist. About 10% local and 90% vocal. We saw a poor devil yesterday who was having a cholecystectomy under a "spinal." His feet were moving and he emitted a terrible groan whenever the professor pulled or cut. The professor injected something into the operation site every so often but it didn't seem to do any good. If it were not for the stoicism of these people, I suspect many would die from shock. Technically, the surgery is all right

since the Japanese are masterful technicians, but the post-op care is quite inadequate.

Japanese buildings are usually one story, rarely more than three (in universities at least). They spread over a large area. Patient laundry hangs in the courtyards and from windows. Experimental dogs are chained to posts in the court immediately outside the wards.

In the afternoon, Professor Kobayashi gave a demonstration to his own class and we saw them in the laboratory. Frogs are used almost exclusively as laboratory animals, although demonstrations are made on mice, rats, rabbits and an occasional dog. Dogs cost 1,000 yen (1/15 the monthly salary of a professor) so not many are used.

Later that afternoon, we attended a tea and reception at Keio University. It has been entirely rebuilt since the war, when it was destroyed by fire. Many professors were there, the president of the University being the host. . . .

Saturday, 19 May 1951, Dai-Ichi Hotel

Yesterday morning I lectured to the students, again on barbiturates. They know nothing about thiopental and were quite impressed by the material. I stayed at the laboratory during the noon hour and chatted with the staff. I was greatly honored by the appearance of Professor Emeritus Hayashi. . . .

Monday, 21 May 1951, Dai-Ichi Hotel

We went yesterday to visit Nikko, 90 miles north of here. We rode to the top of the funicular, took another bus for about a mile, and went down in an elevator several hundred feet to the foot of Kegon Falls which is quite beautiful and resembles Yosemite in some respects. Nikko is at the edge of the mountains and snow-capped peaks are visible close at hand. The azaleas are blooming all over the mountainsides and in gardens. We returned to the shrine area below the funicular and spent all afternoon at the shrine, the most outstanding and beautiful in Japan. It was a magnificent side trip. The shrines are out of this world. . . .

Tuesday, 22 May 1951, Dai-Ichi Hotel

Yesterday's work schedule was lighter than usual. I spent all morning in the pharmacology department, then gave a lecture to the students. We then left and went to Keio University in the afternoon for a clinical pathological conference.

Dr. Kodama (the dean), Professor Kobayashi, myself, and Drs. Ogata, Osawa and Tojo from one of the pharmaceutical houses took the Tokyo group to see the traditional Japanese theater, the Kabuki, which has an all-male cast, the males playing the female parts. It was held in the finest theater in Japan, newly rebuilt after the war. It is a wonderful spectacle of pantomime and symbolism, having an intense emotional appeal. Dr. Hosoya, by bribery of the attendants, arranged to have us visit the principal actor, Utaemon VI, in his dressing room. He was very gracious and permitted us to take pictures of him in the act of making up and being robed in his kimono. He is the sixth member of a theatrical dynasty which goes back over 150 years. It was a delightful experience. I will be terribly hard to get along with when I return home after being so badly spoiled. . . .

Wednesday, 23 May 1951, Dai-Ichi Hotel

Yesterday morning was spent in touring the laboratory of pharmacology with Dr. Kobayashi and his staff. This is the finest department in Japan and they have a fairly large staff. Dr. Kobayashi has about 20 assistants. There are two full professors and two assistant professors. He is connected with a pharmaceutical house and is able to get supplies which most of the laboratories do not have. I feel that they would do good work if they had the money and some training in the U.S. In the afternoon, I gave a demonstration to the students with some new drugs. The students are quite eager for information and some are fairly keen. . . .

Thursday, 24 May 1951, Dai-Ichi Hotel

Yesterday, I gave my last lecture to the students in Tokyo. Professor Kobayashi gave the parting speech afterwards and everything was lovely. I met the dean at Sapporo where we will go. This is on the island of Hokkaido and will be an interesting portion of our trip.

At 4:00 P.M. I went with Professor Maeda, professor of surgery at Keio University and president of the Japanese Surgical Association, his assistant professors, and Dr. Hosoya to see the national wrestling pastime, sumo. Professor Maeda is a consultant for the wrestling association. It was a real spectacle. I was fortunate in being able to see it since it comes to Tokyo for 15 days only twice a year. . . .

Friday, 25 May 1951, Dai-Ichi Hotel

Yesterday morning we had a joint conference with the staff at Tokyo University, discussing American and individual research. The pharmacology group in the Kanto area (Tokyo and environs) gave a special luncheon for me in the department. We then went to the home of Dr. Hosoya. His wife is an M.D. graduate of the Tokyo Women's Medical College. They would like to come to America. They are fine people and I am going to make every effort to get them to Ann Arbor. I was proud to be invited to their home since no others of the mission were afforded that privilege. Dr. Hosoya will be my interpreter in Sapporo and I am delighted to have him with me. In some respects, Japanese civilization is superior to ours. I am struck with their keen intelligence and believe they are worthy of support. . . .

Sunday, 27 May 1951,
Koshien Hotel, Kobe

Fourteen of us left Tokyo by train Saturday evening. We were aroused at 5:00 A.M. and the Kyoto group (Darrow, Soule and Davidson) detrained at 6:50. The Fukuoka group (Volpirro, Johnson, Handler and Miss Snavely) were spending the day in Kyoto and then departing for Kyushu Island. Lucia, Price and Ackerman got off at Osaka and the rest of us (myself, Beeson and Newell) went on to Kobe where we were met by Lt. Colonel Walter with a crew and a weapons carrier to haul our luggage. We were a bedraggled-looking outfit, although the conveniences of the train were not bad.

Are we ever in clover here! We are real VIPs in Kobe. In Tokyo we were not able to compete with all of the generals for the best selections. In Kobe, oh my! We are staying at a lush hotel known as the Koshien, which was a Frank Lloyd Wright design patterned after the Imperial Hotel in Tokyo. It is located 13 miles from Kobe on the way to Osaka. It is a field grade officers' billet for generals and colonels. The commanding general of Southern Japan, stationed in Osaka, lives right above us. Beeson and I have a large sitting room, large bedroom, and a bath looking onto a nice portico. The grounds are lovely and I am sitting here looking onto the gardens with a wandering stream crossed by two typical Japanese red lacquered bridges. We are assigned a car and driver for our personal use and can go anyplace we wish. . . .

Monday, 28 May 1951, Koshien Hotel

This is a really restful place. Last night I had my first good sleep in Japan. This is a gorgeous palace of a hotel which serves both Osaka and Kobe, being about half way between them. We got a leisurely start today and made a courtesy call on the Kobe Base commanding officer, Colonel Roane, at the Shinko Building which contains all of the personnel connected with the base. Kobe is one of the principal military installations in this area. It is a long city lying between Osaka Bay on the south and a ridge of mountains in the north, the city extending way up into the lower foothills where most of the upper class Japanese and nearly all top flight occupation families live, those who came before the ban of last July which prohibits families from coming to this area of Japan. The city was virtually reduced to rubble from bombing and fire but is

being rebuilt rapidly. We had lunch with the Colonel and his aides in the Shinko Building. We can eat in only a few places since virtually all Japanese restaurants are off limits because of unsanitary handling of food.

At 1:00 P.M. we went to the Hyogo Prefectural Medical School, the place where we will be for two weeks. The Medical School is only five years old and was started after the War. They have done quite well in the limited time allotted and have a fairly good faculty. The hospital and Medical School buildings were rebuilt on the framework left standing after the bombing. The hospital houses 500 patients and is dirty, as is usual. In fact, the whole city is dirty, full of rubble and litter in the streets. Our first contact was about our program for the two-week period. This was after an introductory talk by Dr. Shoji, who is 65 and came here to run the new Medical School after retiring at 60 in Kyoto. The usual retirement age is 60 and he is holding on by special dispensation. He is a physiologist and was in Ann Arbor about 1928. We next visited the departments directly since they had planned a reception for us at the Bankers' Club, a very nice modern building. We plan to spend next weekend in Kyoto. It is the sacred city of Japan and was not bombed during the War for this reason. It will be possible to see Japan prewar there. . . .

Thursday, 31 May 1951, Koshien Hotel

On Tuesday, the 29th, we gave a clinical demonstration of two cases with discussions regarding treatment, etc. In the afternoon, I had a conference with the group in pharmacology to plan the program.

On Wednesday, the 30th, I gave two lectures in the morning. About 50 junior and senior medical students and assorted faculty members were in attendance. A staff conference with the pharmacologists of this area (13 medical schools) completed the formal day.

I gave two more lectures to students this morning. This afternoon, I lectured to Japanese pharmacologists without an interpreter who went home with a cold. I hope he is back soon or I will be a flop, although by sign language, writing on the blackboard, etc. we managed to get by. . . .

Sunday, 3 June 1951, Kyoto Hotel, Kyoto

Friday morning we had another joint clinical conference. After lunch, I was picked up by a car from the Takeda Chemical Industries which is located in Osaka only 25 miles from Kobe. My interpreter, Dr. Kumagai, and the professor of pharmacology, Dr. Matsumoto, went with me to visit the Takeda plant. It is the oldest and largest of the pharmaceutical companies in Japan. We arrived in Osaka after a hard trip in a rattletrap car. Practically all of the cars are one to 15 years old and in terrible condition. A large number of cars are wood-burning and have a converter which makes a lot of smoke and stink.

Saturday morning we left on the train to go to Kyoto for the weekend. We were met by a car and taken to the Kyoto Hotel where we were installed in a lovely suite of rooms. Kyoto is the gem city of Japan, the heart of culture. . . .

Monday, 4 June 1951, Koshien Hotel, Kobe

This morning we went to the Medical School where we put on a joint conference. Tomorrow we go to Osaka for the day. We leave here on Friday night to go to Sapporo. . . .

Wednesday, 6 June 1951, Koshien Hotel

Yesterday, we went to Kyoto to shop. There is a museum of old brocades and copies of nearly all the famous ones. In the afternoon, we had a joint conference of the Kobe, Osaka and Kyoto groups.

I gave two lectures this morning and a demonstration this afternoon. This evening Governor Yoshida of the Hyoga Prefecture gave us a dinner. Many dignitaries were present, including Colonel Roane, some foreign office attaches, Mrs. Yoshida, etc. Tomorrow will be the last working day in Kobe. . . .

Friday, 8 June 1951, Allied Train, Kobe to Tokyo

On Thursday, I gave two lectures in the morning. In the afternoon we gave lectures to the Kobe Medical Association.

Today we had a joint clinical conference. After dinner we went to Osaka to board the train for Tokyo where we will take a plane to Sapporo. . . .

Tuesday, 12 June 1951, Grand Hotel, Sapporo

Since arriving in Sapporo, the weather has been rainy and cold. The island of Hokkaido is entirely different from the rest of Japan. In fact, the city of Sapporo was laid out by William Clark, who was the dean of the Massachusetts College of Agriculture in 1876. The streets are straight and the town looks like an American city except for the Japanese influence on types of architecture. The Grand Hotel is the best in Sapporo. We have a corner suite and a bath with a shower, the first one so far.

Sunday we spent the morning wandering about the city. Sapporo is poor compared with the southern cities and very few tourists ever get here.

On Monday we visited the post office. It takes about two extra days to get mail from Tokyo to this area, which is the end of the principal communications. Things are still in short supply since the whole 45th Division of the National Guard troops are located at Camp Crawford and Chitose Air Base. There are many soldiers here as well as the Japanese Home Guard which is being battle-trained under American supervision. This is the northern frontier of Japanese defenses. We were given an official welcome by Vice Governor Fukuda, who is the president of the University and dean of two medical schools here. They have quite a nice auditorium, but the rest of the buildings are very ancient in appearance. In the afternoon, we met with the faculty to make plans for our two-week stay.

After dinner, we attended the puppet

theater. We have been inordinately lucky. We missed the puppet theater in Osaka because they were on tour and then find that they are in Sapporo. It is the Osaka company and probably the best puppeteers in the world. The best known of this company was an 83-year-old man who has been manipulating puppets for 70 years. He was repeatedly decorated by the Emperor. Afterwards, by special arrangement of the governor of Hokkaido, we were taken backstage to meet the actors and have a chance to manipulate the puppets ourselves. It was very interesting and an opportunity afforded few Americans.

Tuesday morning, I lectured for two hours to the students. This afternoon I visited the botanical gardens and greenhouses with Professor Masaki, my counterpart. There is a museum there with Ainu relics. This was of interest since we will visit an Ainu village this weekend. . . .

Friday, 15 June 1951, Grand Hotel

Time has flown by here at a terrific pace. This is the busiest place with continuous activity.

On Wednesday, I gave a staff conference in the morning to the pharmacology department. Thursday morning, I lectured to medical students and in the afternoon attended a clinical pathological conference. I won the grand prize by making the only correct clinical diagnosis from the clinical history and findings. Afterwards, we visited the Hokkaido Industrial Research Institute, a prefectural establishment which is utilizing the natural resources of this area. We were given two unglazed plates on which the Japanese wrote their names and "Japanese American Medical Mission" in Japanese; we wrote our names in English. The plates will be glazed for us to take home.

Friday, I gave a staff conference. We went to the home of the local president of the Rotary club, a great institution in Japan. There is a three day holiday and all of Sapporo is dec-

orated and everyone, including the children, wear their most beautiful costumes. There is a circus in town and in one area is a group of side shows. We got some pictures of the Festival parade which is a parade of the Samurai warriors.

Saturday, we leave in the morning to visit Shirei, an Ainu village and then a famous spa, Noboribetsu. . . .

Wednesday, 20 June 1951, Grand Hotel

On Saturday, we went to Tomakomai, a famous skating center. We had lunch as guests of the Tomakomai Paper Manufacturing Company, which manufactures 80% of the newsprint of Japan. We then went to Shirei. We were taken to the hut of the Miyamoto family of Ainus by Dr. Kodama, professor of anatomy and an authority on the anthropological and ethnological characteristics of the Ainus. We then drove to Noboribetsu where we stayed at the Daiichitakimoto, a Japanese hotel of about 700 rooms, the largest and most famous hotel north of Tokyo. We were put up in the royal suite and were furnished with kimonos which we wore until we left the next day. On Sunday, we left Noboribetsu and drove to Muroran on the Pacific and to Lake Doya to see an active volcano which is called the walking mountain as it rose about 1300 feet above the surrounding plain during a period of three or four years. We then returned to Sapporo.

Monday, there were a lecture and a demonstration in the morning, lunch at the pharmacology department, and a joint conference in the afternoon. We had a formal tea ceremony in a small tea house, which was moved to Sapporo from Kyoto and is a national treasure.

On Tuesday, there was another lecture and a visit to the Franciscan orphanage to see the babies of American fathers and Japanese mothers. In the afternoon, there was a joint lecture and demonstration. We then went to Iwamisawa to give a talk to the local medical society. . . .

6

The University of Michigan Department of Pharmacology with Dr. Seevers 1950–1976: Memoirs of His Administrative Associate

Dorothy H. (Norton) Overbeck, M.A.

My connection with the department began July 1, 1950. At that time, the Department of Pharmacology was small, with just Dr. Seevers, Maynard B. Chenoweth, Gordon K. Moe, Frederick E. Shideman, and Lauren A. Woods. Chen, Gordon, and Fred were associate professors, and Lauren was an assistant professor. Our graduate students were Walter Freyburger under Gordon Moe, Thelma Gould with Fred Shideman, Grace Gray under Dr. Seevers, and Alexander Kandel with Maynard Chenoweth. In the fall of 1950, Walter Freyburger graduated and accepted a position with the Upjohn Company, while Gordon Moe left the department for Syracuse University. Before my arrival, the department had been occupied with World War II projects; even after I arrived, classified projects continued. The department really began to expand in 1951.

I always called Chen, Fred, and Gordon the "Three Musketeers," because they remained close friends until they died. Chen and I kept in touch with annual Christmas letters until his death. Over the years, he mentioned that he, Fred, and Gordon would occasionally get together for reunions. Lauren may have been included in later years, but, in 1950, he was only a junior faculty member. Our professional association was very informal and close-knit. When Dr. Seevers wanted to talk to someone on the third floor, he would not use the telephone. He would walk out into the front hall and yell in a booming voice for a particular faculty member or for one of the graduate students. Lauren, on the first floor, was available for personal walk-in calls. Every afternoon at 3:00 P.M., our old school bell would ring to announce the tea and cookies break. Everyone would gather for a bit of conversation and refreshments as soon as their experiments permitted.

The department had a great deal of money; because of the quality and integrity of our research, Dr. Seevers and his staff had no trouble finding funds. With the addition of more faculty members and the growth in research funds, individual researchers began to acquire their own funding. In 1951, Dr. Seevers journeyed to Japan along with four other faculty members of the University of Michigan. The five of them represented the five basic sciences departments. When Dr. Seevers returned to Ann Arbor, he envisioned an extensive program for the rehabilitation of pharmacology in Japan. He immediately began to search for funds with which to support postdoctoral fellows from Japan.

Eikichi Hosoya was the first Japanese fellow to arrive, in 1952. He found Western culture to be a great challenge, a real foreign phenomenon. I shall never forget his delight when he opened his first checking account and was able to write personal checks. In

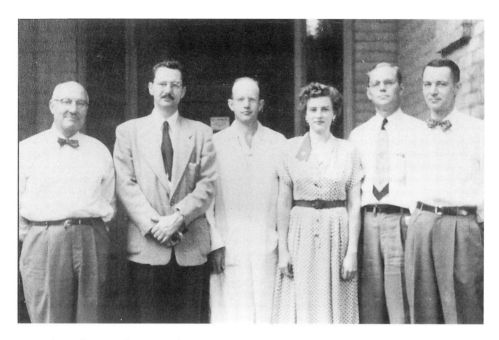

Fig. 1. University of Michigan Pharmacology Department Members, 1951, M. Seevers, M. Chenoweth, M. Nickerson, D. Norton (Overbeck), L. Woods, F. Shideman.

those early years of Japanese fellows, I assisted several of them with their checking accounts. They had to learn how to make bank deposits, balance their checkbooks, and write personal checks.

One of the real dilemmas which Dr. Seevers and I encountered was to try to determine the difference between "yes" and "no." As I recall, there was no such word as "no" in the Japanese language. Even when we knew the answer to a question was no, Eikichi would bow politely and say, "yes." We had to agree with him and then decide which answer was correct. We had the same problem with several of the early Japanese fellows.

One of the most memorable anecdotes I have regarding Eikichi was his purchase of a second-hand automobile. He wanted to drive across the country on a sight-seeing tour from Ann Arbor to California, then sell the car before returning to Japan. He had never driven an American automobile; neither Dr. Seevers nor I knew if he had ever driven one. As I recall, he did a short stint of self-instruction in driving; we were never really certain if he

even acquired a driver's license. Before leaving for California, he was in at least two fender-benders. Dr. Seevers and I were greatly concerned about this trip and were tremendously relieved when he arrived safely in California. I figured he must have had at least 14 guardian angels keeping watch over him.

As time passed, our younger group of Japanese were able to adapt more easily to every aspect of Western customs. Youth gave them the ability to work very diligently, to take advantage of all the opportunities offered them, and to enjoy their introduction to Western society. The most adaptable of all was Tomoji Yanagita. He proved it one day when Mrs. Yanagita and he came strolling into the office. She was fully six feet in front of him with their baby, while Tomoji trailed behind them with her purse in one hand and a teddy bear in the other. When they left, Dr. Seevers and I agreed that the Yanagitas had truly been initiated into American lifestyle.

Akira Sakuma was especially dear to the hearts of all the secretaries. He could create the most wonderful paper birds, animals, etc.

for our pleasure. One time he made some very special ones for one of the girls, who was planning a small party.

One of the most rewarding experiences I had was assisting all of our many foreign students in their desire to improve their English. The Kellogg Foundation routinely sent all of their fellows to the English Language Institute for at least six weeks. We had several serious students who were determined to learn English. The Japanese fellows especially had to spend long hours in studying and speaking.

There were also three non-Japanese who I helped with their English lessons and remember well. Ennio Vivaldi was one of the most serious. I can still picture him with his dictionary in hand, coming down to the office so that we could have our conversation classes on a regular basis. He also wanted to practice telephone conversation. Roberto Vargas had an excellent command of English. He had served an internship in Youngstown, Ohio. He had great trouble with the "w" sound, and was de-

termined to improve his pronunciation. He had the habit of repeating every sentence I would speak to him. Conversation was a slow process, because I, in turn, would correct and comment on his diction. He needed to learn by the repetitive process. Julian Villarreal spoke fluent English. However, when it came to writing letters, he would revert somewhat to Spanish grammar. If he had to write a particularly important letter, he would bring it to me to make corrections. Then we would discuss the grammatical construction.

As I refresh my memory by reviewing the names of all of our former faculty, fellows and graduate students, I find I can remember every one of them. Over those many years, it was my goal to give each and every one special attention and consideration. I had to ruffle some feathers at times, but my heart was always in the right place. Given the opportunity, I would repeat all 27 years with the University of Michigan Department of Pharmacology, working for Dr. Seevers, of course.

Section III.   Japanese Seevers Postdoctoral Fellows: Michigan and Beyond Through the Years

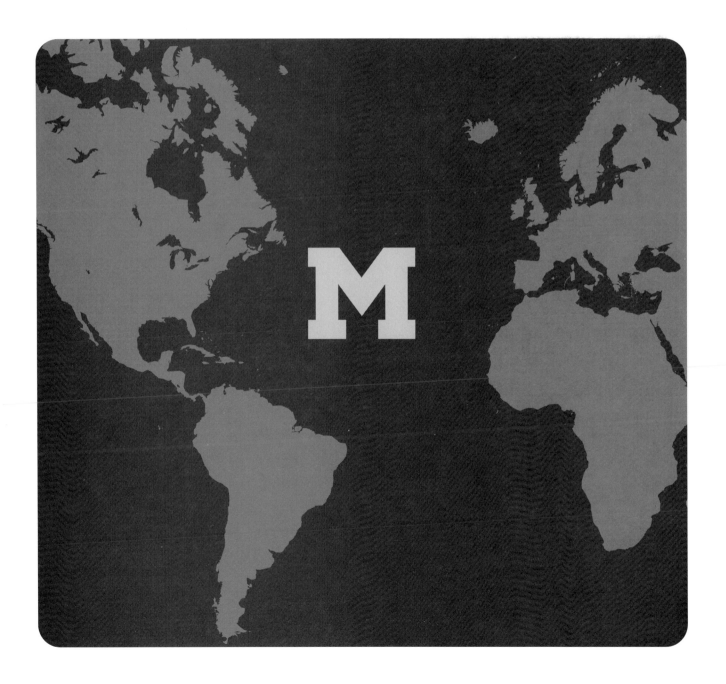

7

Memoir: The Years 1959–1960

Kengo Nakai, M.D., Ph.D.

I studied meperidine metabolism in monkeys under the supervision of Dr. Gerald Deneau. At that time, Dr. Showa Ueki had almost finished up his work in Dr. Domino's lab. He left Ann Arbor soon after my arrival. In spite of my short acquaintance with him, I was deeply impressed by Dr. Ueki and his wonderful personality. He was an energetic person. After he returned to Japan, he devoted his life to studying many different psychoactive drugs.

Dr. A. Sakuma was working in Dr. Lloyd Beck's lab investigating the nature of reflex dilatation in dogs. He displayed an abundance of talent in teaching me statistics, billiards, and how to make spaghetti noodles.

During my stay, I lived in an apartment near North Ingalls Street in Ann Arbor. My place had two rooms so a Japanese friend and I shared the apartment. My first roommate was Dr. Hiroshi Kaneto who studied morphine receptor binding in Dr. Lauren Woods' lab. This became his life's work. We had equal rights and duties in the apartment, and cooked on alternate days. On the days that Hiroshi cooked, everything ran smoothly, but on my days Dr. Kaneto was obliged to eat a lot of uncooked vegetables, such as raw eggplant and fresh spinach. After one such dinner, Hiroshi murmured, "I am not a rabbit." Two weeks later he moved out of the apartment.

My next roommate was Dr. Shuji Takaori from Kyoto who studied the effects of morphine on the CNS in monkeys. On holidays, we frequently played billiards at the Michigan Union. When it was his turn to make dinner, Shuji often prepared Kyoto-style miso soup. I was born in Hokkaido where another type of miso soup is popular. I missed the taste of Hokkaido miso soup so much that I wrote a letter to my wife asking, "Please send me real miso soup as soon as possible."

My last roommate was Dr. Kiro Shimamoto who was Dr. Takaori's senior at Kyoto University. He worked with Dr. Henry Swain. In our apartment, Kiro often enjoyed making instant pickles. It took only two to three minutes to make these salted pickles.

During my stay, which lasted until the summer of 1960, I gradually gained weight. This obesity was the result of the wonderful cooking of all my roommates.

8

Memoir: The Years 1960–1965

◁◇▷

Tomoji Yanagita, M.D., Ph.D.

The 1960s were glorious years for the University of Michigan Department of Pharmacology as well as for the Japanese fellows who studied there. When I arrived in Ann Arbor for the first time in June of 1960, I wondered if I had come to the right place because what was supposed to be a city seemed more like a park with many trees and squirrels. But I soon found that I was indeed in Ann Arbor. Everything was fresh and surprising, including the facilities and equipment which I saw throughout the pharmacology department and the Medical School campus.

When I arrived, my stay overlapped briefly with those of Drs. A. Sakuma, K. Nakai, and H. Kaneto, who left during that year. Dr. S. Takaori was in his second year, and Dr. K. Shimamoto (who was Dr. Takaori's supervisor) joined the group the same year I did. Although the overlap was short, we still had time for some memorable parties with those who were leaving. We benefited greatly from their knowledge of the U.S. as well as of the department. I was greatly impressed when Dr. Sakuma showed me the teaching materials on medical statistics he had prepared for his lectures to postgraduate students. It was hard for me to imagine that any Japanese could teach American postgraduate students after such a brief stay in the U.S. His fishing skills were not quite as impressive. One afternoon, on the way back from the department to the North Campus where I lived, Dr. Sakuma and I walked along the Huron River. He tried to catch a fish there. After hooking a large carp, the line broke and we just missed landing it.

While I was attending the English Language Institute, the instructors taught us not only English but also background knowledge about U.S. life, including such facts as the reason the state of Maine has no medical school (a strong humane society there lobbied against it, objecting to potential animal experimentation), and that the political, business, and academic centers in many states are located in separate cities (a policy based on American philosophy).

After a discussion with Dr. Seevers I decided to undertake dependence studies in the monkey laboratory under the supervision of Dr. G. Deneau, where Dr. Takaori had already spent one year and Dr. Nakai was just finishing up. Although dealing with monkeys was quite a new experience for me, under the guidance and advice of these doctors I was easily able to become accustomed to dealing with Macaca mulatta. Around the same time, Dr. Shimamoto began his work with Dr. H. Swain.

In the 1960s, such faculty members as Drs. L. Beck, D.R. Bennett, T.M. Brody, E.J. Cafruny, E.A. Carr, G.A. Deneau, E.F. Domino, L.B. Mellett, and H.H. Swain were teaching and conducting research under the chairmanship of Dr. Seevers. The department was very active at this time, a reflection of its widely recognized status as the nation's top pharmacology department.

To us Japanese, and perhaps to the rest of the department, Dorothy Norton Overbeck, head administrator of the department, was a most important person. She helped produce documents, and also acted as a liaison with the chairman, transmitting advice to him and so forth. There were two other important department members who cannot be forgotten. One was the boss of the storeroom, Bill Sheldon. We couldn't have obtained any experimental materials without his permission. The department's machinist, Bob Shepherd, was another indispensable member. He constructed all sorts of equipment for the department, and without his cooperation I could never have completed my work. Bob's working hours were 7:30 A.M. to 3:30 P.M. and his invariable reply to requests for equipment construction still rings in my ears: "I'll do it first thing tomorrow morning."

In the monkey laboratory, Dr. Takaori was conducting experiments of electrical stimulation of several brain nuclei, and observed the effects of drugs such as chlorpromazine on physical responses. I made programmable electronic equipment for an avoidance experiment on chlorpromazine, ethyl alcohol, and some sedative hypnotics. I also tried to establish drug self-administration methods, first with oral administration (by drinking) with the animals pressing bars that caused fountain valves to be opened. Ethonitazine, a *mu* agonist resembling morphine but thousands of times more potent, was the first drug I used for oral self-administration. Later, however, we found that oral self-administration has a limitation due to the taste/flavor of certain drug solutions, such as meperidine, which appeared to be aversive to the monkey.

One of the important experiences in studying in a foreign country is having the chance to meet other Japanese who would otherwise be inaccessible. Many Japanese were studying in various departments of the School of Medicine at Michigan, as well as in other non-medical departments. We got together quite often during the evenings and on weekends, not only with the pharmacology colleagues but also with others, sometimes visiting the lakeside or the park for barbecues with our families.

In 1961, Drs. Takaori and Shimamoto left and we welcomed three new Japanese pharmacologists, Drs. S. Iida, T. Furukawa and S. Hisada, all of whom lived in the North Campus apartments. Dr. Iida initiated alcohol studies in the monkey labs. Dr. Furukawa studied the toxic mechanism of CCl_4 in Dr. Brody's lab. Dr. Hisada studied brain amino acids in Dr. Bennett's lab. In the laboratory one day Dr. Iida complained that every day felt like a battle of wits with the monkeys because they were always so talented at destroying his setup.

My self-administration experiments progressed to the intravenous method, and the apparatus for these studies gradually took shape, including attempts to develop the restraining harness. Dr. Seevers was very enthusiastic and supportive of my attempts; Dr. Deneau gave me a lot of good advice. One snowy day, Dr. Deneau took me to Kalamazoo to visit Dr. J.R. Weeks at the Upjohn Laboratories; I learned a lot about catheter techniques from him. Around that time, Dr. A. Wikler, a scholarly psychiatrist-pharmacologist at the Addiction Research Center in Lexington, Kentucky, visited our lab. He was very enthusiastic about our self-administration experiments in monkeys and he talked about what he believed we could learn by using these techniques. He talked and talked the whole afternoon, and seemed as if he were describing his dream for the future. This was an unforgettable experience for me and left me very motivated to accomplish that dream.

In 1962, Dr. Hisada left and Drs. Murano and Akera arrived. Both entered Dr. Brody's lab. Dr. Murano studied $Na^+/K^+/Mg^{++}$ ion-activated ATP-ase. Dr. Akera studied both the biochemical pharmacology of opiate narcotics and ATP-ase. Dr. Murano was always a

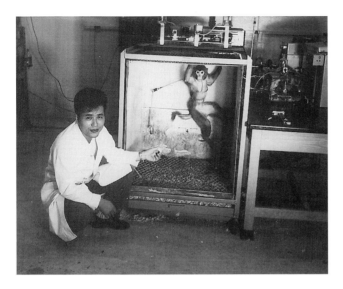

Fig. 1. Dr. T. Yanagita at the UM Pharmacology lab with a new device for self-administration of drugs in a rhesus monkey.

keen discussant of current research issues whenever we Japanese pharmacologists got together. Dr. Akera's long-continued partnership later with Dr. Brody at the Michigan State University Department of Pharmacology was initiated at this time.

In the spring and summer, Drs. Iida, Furukawa, and I often went to play golf at the University or municipal course. Golf was and still is a luxury in Japan and too expensive for young pharmacologists to play. I had to be at the lab even on weekends to refill the drug reservoirs for self-administration experiments and to perform catheter maintenance, but I had enough time in the afternoons to play golf. At that time, I played using golf clubs that had been handed down year to year among the Japanese fellows, starting with Dr. Ueki, who came to the department in 1957 and received the set from Mrs. Seevers. Inasmuch as both Dr. Ueki and myself are rather short, the U.S. women's clubs worked out all right for us. Not only golf clubs, but also various household goods (such as dishes and bowls) were passed along from generation to generation of fellows, usually in pretty tired condition. One reason for this frugality was that, until about 1960, the Japanese were only allowed to take

roughly $50 per person out of the country (this situation improved gradually through the 1960s).

As the development of the self-administration method was progressing well, Dr. Seevers decided to give over the basement (second floor) storage room in Medical Science Building I to self-administration research. Old equipment was discarded, the room was remodeled, and cages were installed by the engineering department. The new lab was completed in late 1962.

I had to give up my Fulbright scholar status (including return trip support) since my stay extended beyond two years. Dr. Seevers instead put me on the teaching staff for the Medical School and postgraduate courses, which allowed me to continue my work.

In February, 1963, the Annual Scientific Meeting of the Committee on Drug Dependence and Narcotics (presently CPDD) was held in Ann Arbor at the Medical School and hosted by Dr. Seevers. My lab was opened for the participants to tour. During that tour, Dr. J.R. Nichols of Southeastern Louisiana College, who was studying self-administration experiments in morphine dependent rats, argued with Dr. N.B. Eddy about the self-administration method as an animal model of psychic dependence. Dr. Nichols' view was based on the belief that drug-seeking behavior is motivated by the withdrawal state, while Dr. Eddy's view (shared by Dr. Seevers) was that drug-seeking behavior can be either based on or independent of the withdrawal state. This discussion continued for longer than two hours while we stood beside the self-administration monkey cages.

One of the most unforgettable events during my stay was the Federation Meeting held in Atlantic City in April, 1963. We Japanese all got together in one motel room and had a sukiyaki party since someone had brought a rice cooker and electric skillet with him. We also bought beer and sake (the sake was a bit deteriorated and had turned dark, but the taste was acceptable). Although the crab and lobster at Hackney's in Atlantic City were justly renowned, the sukiyaki we cooked that night in our room tasted just as good. At the party, Dr. Murano gave a long talk about one of Thomas Mann's novels which impressed the rest of us very much. Later on, however, Dr. Iida sent me that same novel which I found upon reading to be somewhat different from Dr. Murano's version.

In the summer of 1963, Drs. Iida, Furukawa, and Murano left and we welcomed three newcomers, Dr. N. Katsuda, K. Yamamoto and R. Inoki. Both Drs. Katsuda and Yamamoto studied electrophysiologic drug effects in Dr. Domino's lab. Dr. Inoki joined me in the monkey lab to conduct self-administration experiments on nicotine in monkeys for the next two years. After hearing about Japan from these new fellows, I came to realize that the facilities and equipment available there were improving rapidly. They didn't seem as

surprised as I had been when I first saw the department. Around the time of the Tokyo Olympics in 1964, tremendous progress was being made in Japan in many areas.

The members of the department faculty also changed, some leaving, some newly arriving; this was yet another difference from the stable situation in Japanese universities. Every year, when the composition of the Michigan fellows changed, the departmental faculty also changed. Those of us who stayed on always had mixed feelings because it was sad to say good-bye to the friends who were leaving, yet it was also always a pleasure to welcome new faces.

Since my stay became prolonged, I was occasionally summoned by the president of the University or the dean of the Medical School to assist whatever Japanese visitors came. This was a special privilege because I could become acquainted with many famous

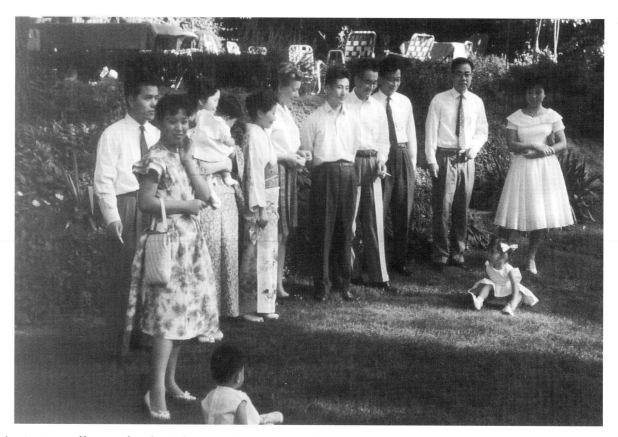

Fig. 2. Farewell party for the Sakumas, Kanetos, and Nakais, and welcome party for the Shimamotos and Yanagitas.

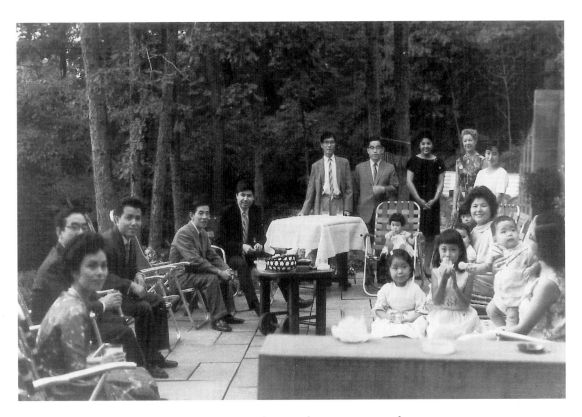

Fig. 3. Group shot in the Seevers' garden.

Japanese professors, university presidents and so on whom I would otherwise never have had the opportunity to meet in Japan. I learned many things from these visitors about Japanese academia and broadened my understanding of scientific knowledge in many fields of medical science, as well as heard from them about what they had seen during their visits to other U.S. universities.

Dr. C.R. Schuster came to the department in 1964 from the University of Maryland to join the self-administration program and to found the operant behavioral laboratory. He added a new sophisticated approach to the drug dependence program in the department.

Every year we enjoyed the departmental and family parties held at Dr. Seevers' home. It was always great fun when he invited all of the Japanese fellows and their families to the various parties held five or six times a year. We enjoyed Mrs. Seevers' cooking as well as Dr. Seevers' hospitality and bartending.

The last year of my stay was 1965. On New Year's Day of 1965, my family invited Dr. Miyata and other Japanese doctors to our apartment for a traditional Japanese-style New Year's dinner, obtaining all of the ingredients from the Japanese food shop in Detroit. By that time, we could get many oriental foodstuffs from the Party Store on Packard Street. In the summer of 1965, Drs. S. Tadokoro and A. Tsujimoto arrived. Dr. Tadokoro joined the monkey labs and studied behavioral pharmacology under Dr. Villarreal. Dr. Tsujimoto was already specialized in the field of nicotine studies and worked on that same issue with Drs. Hudson and Hug.

I was supposed to leave the States due to the Immigration Law as it pertains to exchange scientists. Actually, I was supposed to leave by the summer of 1963, but extended my visa up to the summer of 1964 thanks to Dr. Seevers' letter on my behalf to the Detroit Immigration Office. In 1964, Dr. Seevers again wrote a letter asking to extend my stay for another year. We received no response so I just stayed on. Finally, in May or June of 1965, we were informed that the request had been rejected, but by that time the additional year was practically up anyway. It turned out that I was only able to stay in the U.S. legally for four years, but instead stayed for five years.

When I left the department, the self-administration lab was taken over by Dr. U. Estrada from Mexico and Dr. J.H. Woods, who was a colleague of Dr. Schuster. I believed that my partnership with the monkeys was over for the rest of my research life, and that I would have no chance to revisit the department, but things have turned out quite differently. I was able to establish a monkey lab like Michigan's on my return to Japan, thanks to the strong support of Dr. Seevers. I have visited Ann Arbor and the department almost every year since, a situation which is still continuing to date, some 30 years later.

9

Memoir: The Years 1967–1969

Tetsuo Oka, Ph.D.

It was a privilege for me to have had the opportunity to study pharmacology at the University of Michigan from 1967 to 1969. Since the Department was large, I was able to learn many different aspects of pharmacology. Furthermore Ann Arbor is a beautiful university town and my family (wife and 2 year old daughter) and I enjoyed our lives there. I am grateful to Prof. E. Hosoya who recommended me, Prof. M.H. Seevers who accepted the recommendation, and Dr. C.C. Hug who allowed me to work in his laboratory.

When I arrived at the University of Michigan, three Japanese Pharmacology Fellows had been working there for a year, Dr. Y. Nakai from Kyoto University Faculty of Medicine, Dr. T. Iwami from Hirosaki University School of Medicine, and Dr. M. Miyasaka from Tokyo Medical and Dental University Faculty of Medicine. Dr. M. Matsusaki from Kagoshima University Faculty of Medicine and I began working in September, 1967. A year later, five Michigan Pharmacology Fellows came from Japan, Dr. E. Ikomi from Shinshu University School of Medicine, Dr. T. Fukuda from Kyushu University Faculty of Medicine, Dr. E. Hasegawa from Kyoto Prefectural University of Medicine, Dr. Hitomi from Fujisawa Pharmaceutical Co., Ltd., and Dr. I. Matsuoka from Kyoto University Faculty of Medicine.

Because of the kind arrangements of Professor Seevers and Dr. Hug, I was able to at-tend the meetings of the Federation of American Societies of Experimental Biology in Atlantic City, the meetings of the American Society of Pharmacology and Experimental Therapeutics in Washington, and a narcotic meeting in Indianapolis. At that time, young scientists in Japan usually could not attend such meetings. It was the first time that I was able to attend and I found them to be impressive; they stimulated my scientific interests.

Dr. Hug and his graduate student, J.T. Scrafani, were investigating the uptake of narcotic analgesics into the brain when I joined that project. Dr. Hug had ^{3}H-dihydromorphine (DHM) with quite high specific activity. My interest was directed to the binding of ^{3}H-DHM to opiate receptors in brain tissue. However, the binding of considerable amounts of ^{3}H-DHM to millipore filters made the blank values high and it was not possible to get satisfactory results. After I returned to Keio University in Japan, we could not get ^{3}H-DHM with high specific activity and, therefore, I could not continue such binding experiments. A few years later, Dr. Solomon Snyder and his collaborators got good results by using glass instead of millipore filters. Subsequently, his method was widely employed.

In 1974 (five years after returning to Japan) I moved from Keio University to the Tokai University School of Medicine, which was a new medical school. It is still one of the youngest medical schools in Japan. My new

59

position was Professor and Chairman of the Department of Pharmacology at the recommendation of Prof. Hosoya. At Tokai University, we found that rabbit vas deferens contains *kappa* (κ)-opioid receptors exclusively. By employing this useful isolated preparation, we found that endogenous 6-(Arg or Lys)-opioid peptides such as dynorphins and neo-endorphins were κ-agonists. Recently, we found that the hydrolysis of five endogenous opioid peptides are almost completely prevented by a mixture of three peptidase inhibitors.

After I returned to Japan, over the years I have had the opportunity to see many people associated with the University of Michigan Department of Pharmacology. They were Professor and Mrs. Seevers, Mrs. Overbeck, Professor and Mrs. C. Hug, Professor R. Ruddon and his daughter, Professor H.H. Swain, Professor and Mrs T.M. Brody, Professor and Mrs. E.F. Domino. Professor and Mrs. T. Ueda, and Professor K. Moore. I also met many others from the University of Michigan Department of Pharmacology at various scientific meetings outside of Japan. Among them were Professor J. Woods, Professor S. Holtzmann, Professor J. Villarreal, Professor B. Lucchesi, Professor C. Smith, and Professor T. Tephly. Whenever I see them, I think of the good old days in Ann Arbor.

10

Memoir: The Years 1968–1969

Takeo Fukuda, M.D., Ph.D.

I arrived in Ann Arbor in June of 1968. My first impression was that Ann Arbor was a beautiful and highly civilized city. Living there was far more comfortable than I had expected. I came alone, leaving my wife and children in Japan. I lived in a house at 415 High Street, where many Japanese postdoctoral fellows who came to Ann Arbor without their families lived. On my way to attend the XIIth International Congress of Pharmacology in Montreal, Canada in July of 1994, I visited Ann Arbor again and took a photograph of the front of the house.

When I arrived in Ann Arbor, Drs. K. Matsusaki and T. Oka were in their second year in the department and were working under the supervision of Dr. H. Swain and Dr. C. Hug, Jr., respectively. I attended an eight-week course at the English Language Institute of the University of Michigan with Drs. I. Matsuoka and F. Okomi before starting research work in the department.

At that time in Japan, it was very difficult to use monkeys as experimental animals in pharmacological studies. Therefore, I decided to work in the monkey laboratory under the supervision of Dr. J. Villarreal. I studied the effects of opioids on operant behavior in monkeys. Dr. I. Matsuoka performed electrophysiological studies on vestibular neurons in Dr. Domino's laboratory, and Dr. F. Ikomi studied the reinforcing properties of ethanol in the monkey in Dr. J. Woods' laboratory. In the spring of 1969, Dr. E. Hasegawa came to the department. He lived in the house on High Street and carried out pharmacological studies in Dr. T. Tephly's laboratory.

To study monkeys was a new experience for me. I had to catch a monkey with my hands and set it into a monkey chair before starting my experiments every day. Dr. Villarreal taught me how to handle a monkey but it required a lot of effort for me in the beginning. I implanted stimulation electrodes into

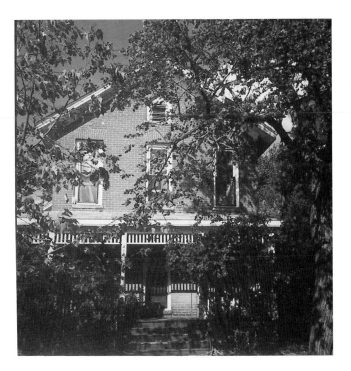

Fig. 1. The house at 415 High Street.

61

monkey brains and started a fixed ratio program. Those experiments were later quite useful in my experimental work in Japan. We are now using the marmoset as an experimental animal in our laboratory.

In the spring 1995 issue of the University of Michigan Pharmacology Department Newsletter, I found an article "In Memorium of Dr. Julian Villarreal." I was deeply shocked to read it. I greatly appreciated his outstanding contributions to opioid dependence research and his warm personality.

11

Memoir: The Years 1980–1985

Tsuneyuki Yamamoto, Ph.D.

As the second Dr. Maurice H. Seevers International Fellow, I arrived in Ann Arbor on April 1, 1982, when it was covered with snow. My family and I were astonished and speechless to see the cold snowscape. We had not expected such heavy snow in April. The snow was still falling thick and fast on the night we arrived. Looking through the car window, I had some uneasy and anxious feelings about our future in Ann Arbor. At that time, I couldn't have known that warm spring was already waiting to come out from under the wintry snow.

By the time I arrived, Dr. Naohisa Fukuda, a research scientist at the Central Research Division of Takeda Pharmaceutical Co., Ltd., had been studying the effect of phencyclidine in rhesus monkeys in Dr. Ed Domino's laboratory since August, 1981. It seemed that he had already become a good American.

My research themes, assigned by Dr. James Woods, were diuresis produced by *kappa* opioids in rhesus monkeys, and drug discrimination on serotonergic compounds in pigeons. I could demonstrate in the former the diuretic effect of the *kappa* agonist U-50488 at µg/kg doses. With the latter research, two classes of 5-HT recognition sites, namely, 5-HT_1 and 5-HT_2, had been identified using radioligand binding studies. I tried to elucidate whether pigeons trained to discriminate the 5-HT_1 (1-5-HTP), and 5-HT_2 (quipazine) agonists, respectively, from saline, might provide

useful information on differentiating the effects of compounds with diverse serotonergic profiles. The results demonstrated the usefulness of the method to clarify the functional aspects of receptor subtypes as well as agonist/antagonist interactions among serotonergic compounds. After I left Ann Arbor, the diuresis and discrimination studies were respectively taken over by Dr. Debra Gmerek, who moved to Warner Lambert several years later, and Dr. Ellen Walker, then a postgraduate student, now in Dr. Alice Young's lab at Wayne State University.

At the end of April, 1983, Dr. K. Takada, a researcher at the Preclinical Research Division of the Central Institute for Experimental Animals, came to Ann Arbor. His research was focused on the mechanism mediating aversive and anxiogenic effects of drugs; collaborating with Dr. Gail D. Winger, he trained pigeons to discriminate bemegride from saline. He also trained rhesus monkeys to terminate intravenous infusion of histamine, and further to discriminate the effect of ethyl ß-carboline-3-carboxylate (βCCE), an inverse agonist at the benzodiazepine receptor, from saline, in a different group of monkeys. He could demonstrate the aversive property of *kappa*-agonists after repeated exposure to drugs. He showed that the discriminative effect of βCCE was anxiogenic in nature. These results delighted him and gave him an anxiolytic state, it seemed. He also conducted some pigeon experiments. When either of us got nice data, or when we had had a bad day, or, really, whenever we felt like it, we further worked on "alcohol dependence" clinical studies after we left the lab, going out drinking until late at night. Dr. Takada spent two years in Ann Arbor and then another year at the Addiction Research Center, now the Intramural Division of NIDA, returning to Japan in 1986.

In Dr. Woods' lab, "lab meetings" were held weekly on the research being undertaken; each member gave a progress report followed by a group discussion. The meetings lasted at least a couple of hours. The discussion was very aggressive and uninhibited in that everybody in the lab, including not only postgraduate students such as Dr. Charles P. France, now a professor of pharmacology at Louisiana State University, but even high school kids who were running pigeon experiments, uttered their opinions freely, regardless of their scientific background. This was very novel to me because in Japan we choose only to listen when the subject or field is not familiar to us. In order to mingle with the atmosphere, I tried early during the meetings to utter several questions, before I became deaf and mute to English by exhaustion from con-

centrating to catch what was going on. I believe each session worked very well. If you had no new data to present at the meeting, you had to rack your brain to produce some scientific excuse no matter how lame it was. Other than the lab meetings, there was a yearly joint meeting with Dr. C.R. Schuster's lab at the University of Chicago, which alternated in Chicago and Ann Arbor. In Dr. Schuster's lab, experiments on the subjective effects of drugs in humans were conducted, in addition to the animal experiments. It was very interesting and informative because experimental drug studies in humans were rare in Japan.

Apart from scientific work, there were several memorable events held in Ann Arbor. On May 29, 1982, the 9th Annual Dexter-Ann Arbor Run was held with over 1,000 people participating. Dr. Woods, his lab staff (including Dr. J.L. Katz, who became my marathon coach, and is now at the Division of Intramural Research of NIDA) and I attended a 10 km (6.2 mile) run from Delhi Metropark to downtown Ann Arbor. Although I placed 146th in the 30–34 age group (time: 52 min, 46 sec), I can proudly say that I was the number one Japanese runner (note: no other Japanese entry)!

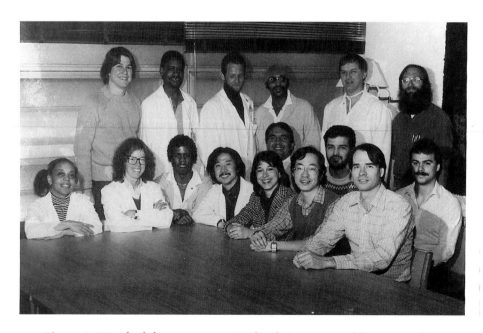

Fig. 1. A Woods' lab meeting in Medical Science Building I in 1982.

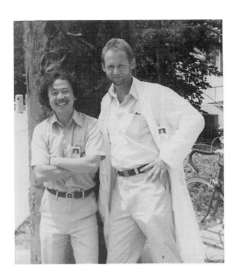

Fig. 2. Drs. T. Yamamoto and C.P. France in front of the sculpture by the Taubman Medical Library.

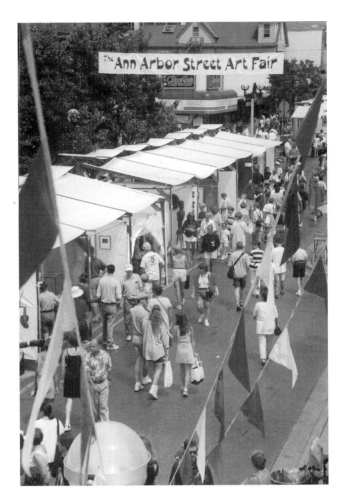

Fig. 3. A street scene of the Ann Arbor Art Fair in July.

Another big annual event in Ann Arbor is the Ann Arbor Art Fair. As the 3rd week of July rolls around, Ann Arbor residents close off to vehicle traffic many streets, like South and North University, State, Liberty, Maynard, and Main Streets, so that artists and craftsmen can open stalls to exhibit and sell their works. People are awash in the streets. It became a year-marker for me as the turning point of summer. I am a woodcarving artist as well as a pharmacologist; I was busy but enjoyed every minute of this period. It was like "even when the cats are there, mice will go to the Art Fair."

In 1984, my family and I left Ann Arbor. My heart was too full for words. Although the winter in Ann Arbor had been very severe, we felt so warm when we left Ann Arbor for Japan. It is unforgettable indeed. We are still grateful that Mrs. Seevers treated us as though she had adopted us. She always laughed at my poor jokes and made my family feel at home in every possible way. I just cannot imagine our Michigan life without her.

I had a chance to join Dr. Woods' lab again in 1988 as an exchange researcher of the Naito Foundation for three months. I had two research themes during the second visit. One was to clarify the discriminative stimulus

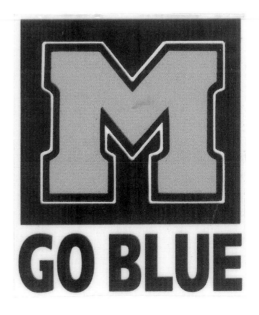

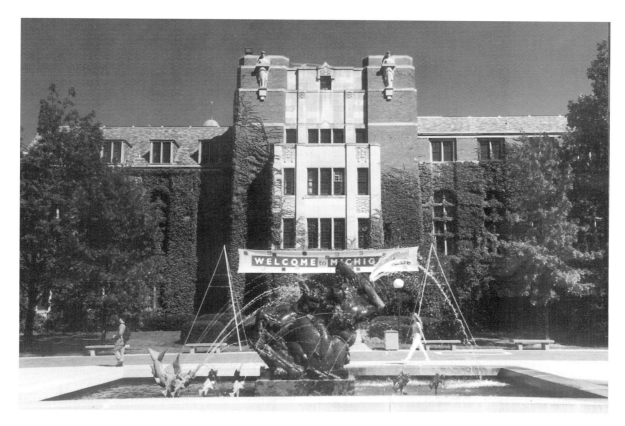

Fig. 4. A view of the Michigan League and its fountain in the foreground in September.

properties of βCCE in the pigeon, and the other was to establish a method to measure respiratory and ventilation rates in unanesthetized rhesus monkeys. During the course of the latter study, I demonstrated the respiratory depressant effect induced by μ-opioid agonists.

In Japan, I continued research on the discriminative effects of novel compounds such as an atypical anxiolytic tandospirone, a NMDA antagonist dextrorphan, the cholinesterase inhibitors THA and amiridine, and an OTC cough cure solution "Bron." Since the drug discrimination procedure was not very popular in Japan, a few scientists of the field, including Dr. Takada and me, founded the Drug Discrimination Study Group in 1988. The study group held annual meetings for six

years which gathered about 80 young scientists every year. In recent years, my research focus has been on mechanisms underlying learning and memory using an operant conditioning procedure which I learned at the University of Michigan.

Mrs. Seevers passed away on March 21, 1993, and my boss, Dr. Showa Ueki, followed her on June 22nd. My family and I were saddened and overshadowed with the sorrow of losing two of our dear friends in such a short period of time.

Beyond spatial and temporal phases, I can still hear the cheerful sounds of "Hail to the Victors" and see the maize and blue of the University of Michigan whenever I close my eyes.

12

Memoir: The Years of 1985–1986

Masaru Minami, M.D., Ph.D.

In 1984, Dr. Tsuneyoshi Tanabe told me to contact Dr. H. Swain, then an assistant dean, concerning the possibility of doing research at the University of Michigan. Dr. Swain, always sincere, kindly wrote a letter to Dr. Tanabe. In his letter, he said that Dr. B. Lucchesi had looked at my curriculum vitae and would offer me a fellowship for the following year in his laboratory. I fortunately got a 10 month official foreign trainee position from September, 1985 to June, 1986 that was financially supported by the Japanese Ministry of Education. I was told more about Dr. Lucchesi's laboratory by Dr. Akira Ueno of the Nagasaki University School of Medicine, who had spent several weeks in Dr. Lucchesi's laboratory in September and October of 1983. I also asked Dr. T. Yamamoto, on the faculty of pharmaceutical sciences at Kyushu University, about the Department of Pharmacology at the University of Michigan.

I arrived in September, 1985. At that time, there were no Japanese fellows in the Department of Pharmacology. Dr. Joe Linch met me upon my arrival at Detroit Metropolitan Airport and kindly assisted in getting me oriented to the laboratory and Ann Arbor. While I stayed in Ann Arbor, I lived in the Island Drive Apartments along the Huron River. It was a five minute walk to Medical Science Building I from my apartment. Furthermore, the Island Drive Apartments were located very close to Japanese and Korean food markets.

In the autumn of 1985, Dr. Nobuyuki Morisaki, of the Yamagata University School of Medicine, joined us with his wife, Dr. Junko Morisaki. They were studying the drug response to the isolated uterine smooth muscle, and stayed at the Women's Hospital in the Medical Center as gynecologists. Dr. Morisaki and I got together quite often in the evenings and on weekends, visiting Japanese restaurants and exploring beyond Ann Arbor using Dr. Morisaki's Honda. Dr. Morisaki later opened a maternity clinic in Sakata City, Yamagata Prefecture.

In 1985, Drs. J. Linch, S. Werns, C.V. Jackson, P. Simpson et al. were conducting research with Dr. Lucchesi. My project was to evaluate the cardiovascular effects of BMY21190, an inhibitor of cAMP phosphodiesterase. E. Driscoll kindly assisted my experiment using the canine model of coronary artery thrombosis. Dr. Lucchesi was very active in and supportive of my project. During my stay in Michigan, I wrote eight reports. With permission of the drug company, I have published the reports in four scientific papers: *Cardiovascular Drug Reviews, Japanese Circulation Journal, Pharmacology,* and *Biogenic Amines.* More than 10 years after returning to Japan, I can still demonstrate the evidence that I studied under Dr. Lucchesi.

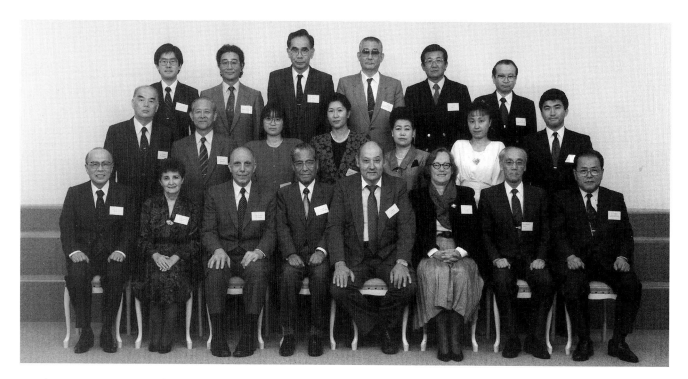

Fig. 1. Participants of the Japanese Michigan Fellows meeting and buffet, September 21, 1990, Sapporo, Japan.

I have learned many things from visitors to the Lucchesi laboratory via discussions with them. Every evening after the visitors' lectures, Dr. and Mrs. Lucchesi invited me to dinner. I enjoyed very much the dinners at Italian restaurants as well as Mrs. Lucchesi's cooking in their home. In September 1990, Drs. Tanabe, Yanagita, Saito, my supervisor, and I invited Dr. and Mrs. Lucchesi to Sapporo as a guest speaker at the scientific meeting for the Japanese Association of Clinical Pharmacology. In addition to Dr. and Mrs. Lucchesi, Dr. and Mrs. Domino were hosted by the Michigan fellows at a pleasant evening buffet. It was especially nice to see the number of wives who attended, making the occasion a truly memorable one. Dr. Tanabe, who had been the second Japanese fellow at the University of Michigan, was very active as host.

In the winter of 1985, Dr. Masanori Senjo, a psychiatrist from Hokkaido University School of Medicine, spent several weeks in the Department of Pharmacology as a visiting scholar sponsored by the Japanese Ministry of Education. In April, 1986, he became an asso-

ciate professor of clinical psychology at the Health Sciences University of Hokkaido. At around the same time, Dr. Iwao Saito, one of my colleagues, visited Dr. Lucchesi's laboratory. In 1991, he became a professor at Muroran Institute of Technology, in Hokkaido. After my return to Japan in October, 1986, I moved from Hokkaido University and have succeeded the chair of Dr. Tanabe in the Department of Pharmacology at the Health Sciences University of Hokkaido.

From Sapporo, Hokkaido, Dr. Mitsuhiro Yoshioka, Hokkaido University School of Medicine, joined Dr. C.B. Smith's laboratory and studied neuropharmacology. Later, Dr. Toru Endo, of the Health Sciences University of Hokkaido, studied in Dr. Smith's laboratory.

I am very appreciative of Drs. Swain, Lucchesi and Smith for their help during my stay in Ann Arbor. What I learned and worked on in the Department of Pharmacology at the University of Michigan has made me happy and self-confident.

13

Memoir: The Years 1989–1990 and Beyond

Mitsuhiro Yoshioka, M.D., Ph.D.

In the summer of 1989, I joined a glorious family in the Department of Pharmacology at the University of Michigan as a Maurice H. Seevers International Fellow. As a cardiovascular pharmacologist in Japan, I had been studying serotonergic mechanisms in the regulation of blood pressure in the central nervous system. My supervisor, Professor Hideya Saito, who chaired the First Department of Pharmacology at Hokkaido University School of Medicine from 1975 to 1997, recommended me as a candidate for the Seevers Fellowship. Professor Emeritus Tsuneyoshi Tanabe, the second Japanese fellow at Michigan from 1957 to 1959, also recommended me. Unfortunately, Professor Tanabe passed away in the winter of 1996. Because of their fine recommendations, I received the Fellowship and joined the laboratory of Dr. Charles B. Smith.

When I arrived in Ann Arbor, this being my first trip to the United States, a funny event occurred. I needed U.S. dollars to buy some McDonald's hamburgers but I had only travelers checks. Since I wanted to exchange my travelers checks for cash, I went to a nearby bank. I think it was First of America across from the Medical Science Building I. I asked a beautiful young clerk, "Please cash my fifty dollar travelers check?" She replied with a smile, "How would you like it?" I could not understand her meaning at that time but I felt compelled to say something as quickly as possible. I hesitated briefly and then replied, "I like it very much." The result of my answer is easy to figure out with no explanation. I should have said, "In five ten dollar bills, please." That was the reason I attended the English Language Institute to improve my knowledge of the subtleties of the English language.

In the laboratory of Dr. Smith, I continued my studies of serotonergic mechanisms in the central nervous system. He and his colleagues had shown previously that drugs and treatments used to treat melancholia and a variety of other psychiatric disorders decrease the density of α_2 adrenoceptors located in specific areas of the rat brain. Such drugs produce a functional subsensitivity of those receptors that regulate the release of norepinephrine from both neurons in the rat brain and from peripheral noradrenergic neurons in the rat heart. During the year that I worked with Dr. Smith, we demonstrated that α_2 receptors located on serotonergic neurons in the hippocampus and the dorsal raphé nucleus of the rat brain also regulate the release of 5-hydroxytryptamine (serotonin). These kinds of effects are critical areas of further contemporary pharmacological research in both the peripheral and the central nervous system. Hence, I spent a most valuable period of training.

At that time, Dr. Raymond Ruddon was the Chairman of the Department of Pharmacology at Michigan, but he was leaving shortly to become head of the Eppley Cancer Institute at the University of Nebraska Medical Center in Omaha. When Dr. Hosoya and his wife came to Ann Arbor in the autumn of 1989, I joined Dr. Ruddon, Dr. James Woods and Dr. Henry Swain at the home of Mrs. Seevers for a wonderful visit during which time we chatted with Dr. Hosoya. I felt fortunate to be asked to share this occasion with such VIPs.

During my stay in Ann Arbor, I carried for my lunch onigiri, which is made of steamed rice and is a very common component of a Japanese lunch. Usually, I ate onigiri with miso soup, which is also a very traditional Japanese dish. I recall that every lunchtime the atmosphere of our laboratory took on a Japanese aroma. I did not know whether my colleagues liked it or not.

After returning to Japan, I kept in touch with Dr. Smith for many years. In 1992, Dr. Smith received a Japan Society for the Promotion of Science (JSPS) Fellowship for Research in Japan. The JSPS Fellowship for Research in Japan was established in 1959 to promote international cooperation and mutual understanding in scientific research. This program is supported by a Japanese government subsidy and is designed to enhance contacts between scientists in Japan and other countries, a condition favorable to the promotion of future scientific cooperation and exchange.

During his stay in our laboratory in Sapporo, Dr. Smith conducted a project using the technique of *in vivo* microdialysis in which a dialysis probe is inserted stereotaxically into the hippocampus of the awake, unrestrained rat. This study provided the first demonstration that an antidepressant drug causes a subsensitivity of α_2 adrenoceptors on serotoner-

gic neurons in the rat brain *in vivo*. This finding is similar to that observed previously for α_2 adrenoceptors on noradrenergic neurons in a variety of *in vitro* preparations. Other experiments conducted during Dr. Smith's visits to Sapporo were related to the characterization of opioid receptors that regulate the release of 5-hydroxytryptamine from rat hippocampus neurons during *in vivo* microdialysis. These studies involved the use of agonists and antagonists highly specific for μ-, κ-, and δ-opioid receptors. The data indicate that the μ-opioid receptor is the predominant opioid receptor that regulates neuronal release of serotonin in the hippocampus of the rat.

In the spring of 1997, Dr. Smith organized a symposium entitled "Interactions of Neuronal Systems at Presynaptic Receptors" at the Pharmacology '97 meeting in San Diego, California in honor of my superior, Professor Hideya Saito. This symposium was held under the auspices of the Neuropharmacology Division of the American Society for Pharmacology and Experimental Therapeutics. Dr. Peggie J. Hollingsworth edited the proceedings of the symposium. Her talents always surprised us and were very valuable.

All of these events are unforgettable for not only Professor Saito but also for all of the members of our department. The collaboration that now exists between our group in the First Department of Pharmacology at the Hokkaido University School of Medicine and that in the Department of Pharmacology at the University of Michigan Medical School has been strengthened greatly. I look forward to years of future productive collaboration and to the exchange of scientists and scientific information between our two departments.

14

Memoir: The Years 1993–1995

Shin-ichi Iwata, M.D., Ph.D.

I was in Ann Arbor from September, 1993 to June, 1995. Together with my wife, Mikayo, and our 2 year old son, I flew from Narita International Airport, looking forward with pleasure and anxiety to my stay in the United States. After a 14 hour flight, we arrived at Detroit Metro Airport where we were met by Dr. Margaret Gnegy, a famous researcher in calmodulin and amphetamine sensitization. Thus began our unforgettable stay in Ann Arbor. Denise Gakle, an Administrative Associate in the Department of Pharmacology, made a reservation for us at a hotel in Ann Arbor where we had to settle ourselves for a week. We then rented an apartment in the Willow Tree Complex. We had a really good backyard and a broken oven which no one could fix. We were there for a year, then moved to another apartment complex. We opened a bank account, first rented then later bought a car, and made all of our arrangements for a stay in Ann Arbor. We bought a vacuum cleaner which was the only one we could find. Later we realized that this type of vacuum was meant to be used in the basement or outside the house. It made a huge noise. We have to give special thanks to Yasuko Ueda, the wife of Dr. Ueda, a Professor of Pharmacology and Psychiatry. She taught us to live in the U.S. and was very helpful in getting us settled in Ann Arbor.

There were nine people in the laboratory of Professor Gnegy. All of the others were studying calmodulin using cultured cells. I devoted myself to *in vivo* and *in vitro* amphetamine sensitization studies in rats. We presented the results of our research in turn every Friday, providing a good opportunity to study different fields of knowledge.

There was one other postdoctoral fellow working in the lab, Zia Madar, an Iranian. His wife, Fakri, sometimes helped my wife at the Modern Montessori Nursery School where her son, Bahbak, and my son, Tomoyuki, were enrolled. Mikayo was not fluent in

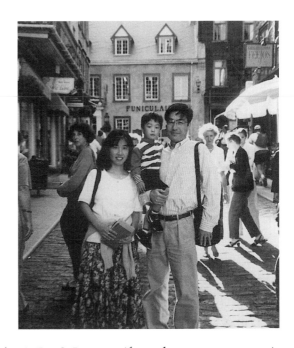

Fig. 1. Dr. S. Iwata, wife, and son on an auto trip to Quebec City, Canada.

71

English and had difficulty communicating with the teachers. During our stay, she found many friends in Ann Arbor. Tomoyuki needed friends of his age so Mikayo had to find friends for him.

There were three postgraduate students in the lab, Adam, Sharon, and Kim. Adam was the most senior of the three and helped keep the lab in order. He always said "don't forget to turn off the light" and "the computer in the lab should be shut down in an appropriate way." Keiki was a research associate in the lab and we sometimes worked together. We got our lunches from a greasy food restaurant, Angelo's, which helped me gain 6 pounds during my stay in the U.S. I still miss the chili from Angelo's. Keiki taught me many English phrases and words, including slang. Her husband, Skip, worked in the music world. Keiki took Mikayo to an REM concern in Detroit, which was a precious experience for her.

Dr. Gnegy had a lab party each summer and a Christmas party each year. Her house was in a suburb of Ann Arbor and had a pond in the backyard with several swans. She was a good cook. Her lasagnas were excellent. Dr.

Gnegy's husband, Wes, was a cultured person. The first time I conversed with him, I could not understand him very well. I felt like I was reading the Times. However, when they visited Kagoshima in the fall of 1997 he used easy English words to talk with us.

We made many Japanese friends in Ann Arbor. I believe there were more than 40 Japanese working in the Medical Center. Dr. Toku Takahashi, an Assistant Research Scientist in the Department of Gastroenterology, organized a Japanese get-together. He gave a year end part in a Japanese restaurant. Many Japanese were working in automobile companies in Ann Arbor and also in the Department of Technology. A famous Japanese professor worked in this department and many of the Japanese employed by Japanese automobile companies studied in the lab.

In 1994, the Department of Pharmacology moved to a new building. Fortunately, our lab had windows but underground rooms were allotted to several other labs. The Department also got a new chairman in 1994, Dr. Paul Hollenberg.

I would like to describe my research in

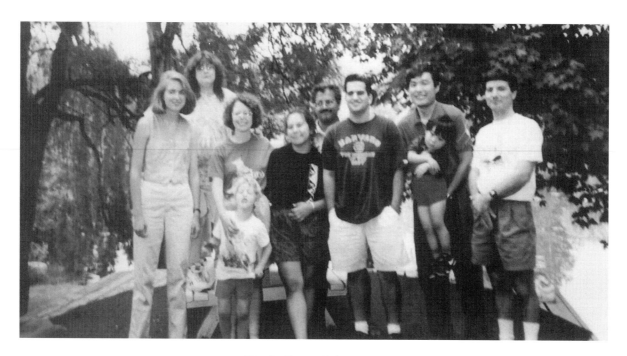

Fig. 2. Gnegy lab party.

Dr. Gnegy's lab. Amphetamine is a psychomotor stimulant which is a serious addiction problem in Japan and the U.S. Repeated doses of amphetamine induce sensitization to the drug. Investigations using laboratory animals have revealed that the expression of sensitization is due to the enhanced release of dopamine caused by an accelerated phosphorylation of synapsin I by the activation of calmodulin kinase II (CKII). Synapsin I is a vesicle-related protein modulating the release of classical transmitters. In sensitized animals, we also found an increase of phosphorylated neuromodulin which is a multifunctional protein related to transmitter release, development, regeneration, plasticity, etc. In a separate experiment, we showed that low doses of amphetamine enhanced phosphorylation of synapsin I site 3 in synaptosomes and that this enhancement was inhibited, in part, by D_1 receptor antagonists and PKC inhibitors, although synapsin I site 3 is phosphorylated through CKII. Dr. Gnegy was invited to be a lecturer at the 27th Annual Meeting of the Japanese Society of Neuropsychopharmacology held October 21–22, 1997 in Kagoshima. At that time, she presented the results mentioned above. Many Japanese pharmacologists and psychiatrists are interested in amphetamine and methamphetamine sensitization so they were impressed by her lectures.

My family and I had a very enjoyable time in Ann Arbor. I am appreciative to the members of the Japanese Michigan alumni and Dr. Gnegy. I had a very productive experience at the University of Michigan.

15

Memoir: The Years 1995–1997

Shiroh Kishioka, M.D., Ph.D.

I joined the Department of Pharmacology as a Maurice H. Seevers International Fellow in September, 1995. I was a staff member in the laboratory of Dr. James H. Woods. When I arrived at Detroit Metro Airport, Dr. Gail Winger, who is Mrs. Woods, was waiting just outside the Customs area of the airport carrying a name board with my name on it. I immediately saw her and she took me to Ann Arbor. Dr. Edward F. Domino had arranged my housing at Baits House student dormitory on the North Campus and I stayed there for a few days. Thus, my fruitful life in Ann Arbor started.

At that time, most of the Department of Pharmacology laboratories and equipment had moved into Medical Science Research Building III. However, Dr. Woods' laboratory was still in Medical Science Building I. Dr. Woods was interested in *in vivo* behavior in mice, rats, pigeons and monkeys and these animals were housed in MSB I. In particular, there were 130 rhesus monkeys which were used for experiments. My office was also located in MSB I. Since there were no windows in Dr. Woods' laboratory, we could not tell what the weather was like until we went outside. I had heard that Dr. Seevers had been the supervisor of Dr. Woods and that his office had been in this building. Dr. Woods still kept a commemorative plaque for Dr. Seevers at the entrance to his office.

Lab meetings were held at noon for one hour Monday through Friday unless we attended seminars or Dr. Woods was out of town. At each lab meeting, two or three of the lab members presented their data and we all discussed the results. More than 20 members were part of Dr. Woods' laboratory including postgraduate students, pre- and postdoctoral fellows, and research investigators.

In January, 1996, I started research on opioid effects on respiration using seven rhesus monkeys. The experimental techniques for the assessment of respiratory function in the monkeys was already in place in Dr. Woods' laboratory. During my initial studies, I tried to elucidate the agonist and antagonist properties of new opioid compounds, as estimated by respiratory functions in rhesus monkeys. In the studies that followed, I tried to assess the monkeys' acute dependence on morphine and heroin because I had been studying acute opioid dependence in rodents in the Department of Pharmacology at Wakayama Medical College in Japan. Dr. Woods was also interested in acute dependence. After we assessed acute opioid dependence using respiratory functions, we examined the effects of N-methyl-D-aspartate antagonists and an L-type calcium channel blocker, both of which were well known as suppressants of opioid withdrawal. We studied their effects on opioid antagonist induced withdrawal, as estimated by respiratory function. During these experiments, we found that an L-type calcium channel blocker could dissociate morphine-induced analgesia and respiratory suppression; that is, the calcium channel blocker enhanced the analgesic but not the respiratory depressant effects of morphine. Our results were presented at the meetings of the European Behavioral Pharmacology Society '96 held in Cagliari, Italy in May, 1996; the 58th College on Problems of Drug Dependence in San Juan, Puerto Rico, June, 1996; the 27th International Narcotic Research Conference held in Long Beach, California, July, 1996; the 59th College on Problems of Drug Dependence, held in Nashville, Tennessee, June, 1997; and the 28th International Narcotic Research Conference, held in Hong Kong, August, 1997. These presentations were excellent training for me.

Since I came to Ann Arbor alone, leaving my family in Japan, I rented a one bedroom apartment at the Medical Center Court. I liked the view from the window of my apartment since I could see the entire University of Michigan Medical Center. The apartment was a very convenient 15 minute walk from the laboratory and was also close to a supermarket, Krogers, an oriental grocery, Manna, a pizza house and a restaurant. My family visited Ann Arbor in August, 1996 and March, 1997. During those times, we went to Detroit, Niagara Falls, Toronto, Chicago, Orlando, New York and the lower peninsula of Michigan. The memory of our trips in the U.S. will live with us forever.

Drs. Woods and Winger often took the staff, including me, to various kinds of restaurants i.e., Japanese, Chinese, German, Italian, American, etc. On Thanksgiving Day of every year, they held a party in their home and invited the staff of their laboratory. Dr. Winger cooked a turkey and other foods and Dr. Woods served them to everyone. I particularly remember the pumpkin pie, which was served as dessert. Just before I left Ann Arbor, Drs. Woods and Winger held a farewell party for me in their home and all of the staff participated in the party.

From May 31 to June 2, 1996, Dr. Tetsuo and Mrs. Oka visited in Ann Arbor just before going to the FASEB '96 meetings. Dr. Oka is a Professor in the Department of Pharmacology, Tokai University School of Medicine. He lived in Ann Arbor from 1967 to 1969 when he was a member of the staff of the Department of Pharmacology. During their visit Dr. and Mrs. Oka went to North Campus to see the residence where they had lived 28 years before. They found the apartment and were reminded of the good old days. They also had dinner with Drs. Woods and Winger at the Bell Tower Hotel.

I completed my postdoctoral appointment in Pharmacology in May, 1997. After my return to Japan, I resumed my position in the Department of Pharmacology at Wakayama Medical College. I am very grateful to Drs. Woods and Winger, as well as all of the staff in Dr. Woods' laboratory and the Department of Pharmacology, the Maurice H. Seevers International Fellowship in Pharmacology, and, in particular, to the members of the Japanese Michigan alumni.

Just before I left Ann Arbor, Miss Sayaka Yamamoto, the daughter of Dr. Tsuneyuki Yamamoto, stayed in Ann Arbor for several months in order to study English. She stayed at University Towers where she had lived with her father several years before. During her stay in Ann Arbor, she visited the offices of Dr. Domino (he put her to work) and Dr. Woods. She also joined my farewell party.

I have also heard of other Japanese people who studied in the Department of Pharmacology at the University of Michigan. Dr. Miki Takasuna was one of them. Dr. Takasuna joined the Woods' laboratory in the fall of 1991. She was introduced to Dr. Woods by Dr. Kohni Takada who studied in Dr. Woods' laboratory from 1983 to 1985. Her project was on the opioid pharmacology of the antinociceptive effects of loperamide. After completing her research project in Ann Arbor, she resumed her position in the Department of Psychology at the University of Tsukuba. Her present position is in the Psychology Laboratory at Yamano College of Aesthetics.

From April to June 1996, Dr. Hiroko Togashi worked in the laboratory of Dr. Charles B. Smith. She studied 5-HT releasing mechanisms mediated by *kappa* opioid receptors in rat hippocampus. I heard that she had a fruitful time in Ann Arbor, despite a short stay. Her present affiliation is in the First Department of Pharmacology at the Hokkaido University Graduate School of Medicine

Dr. Katsuharu Saito of the Department of Internal Medicine at Hokkaido University School of Medicine, and Dr. Kumi Saito of the Department of Ophthalmology at Sapporo Medical University arrived in Ann Arbor in August, 1996. They joined the laboratory of Dr. Benedict R. Lucchesi. Dr. K. Saito studied

not only in Dr. Lucchesi's laboratory but also at the Kellogg Eye Center. They returned to Japan in August, 1997.

Outside the Department of Pharmacology, from April, 1991 to September, 1992 Dr. Hiroshi Ueda studied in the laboratory of Dr. Daniel Goldman, who was affiliated with the Mental Health Research Institute. Dr. Ueda is now a Professor in the Department of Molecular Pharmacology and Neuroscience at the Nagasaki University School of Pharmaceutical Sciences.

Over 40 Japanese researchers studied the medical sciences at the University of Michigan Medical School. From 1992, we held a private Japanese Circle in the Medical Center, organized by Dr. Toku Takahashi of the Department of Gastroenterology, where seminars were held on Fridays every two months.

16

Seevers Fellows' Activities in Japan

◄○►

Tomoji Yanagita, M.D., Ph.D.

Western medical science was brought to Japan by the Dutch during the Edo Era (the 1770s). When the modernization of Japan began in earnest in the Meiji Era (the 1870s), medical science developed rapidly following the model of German medicine; this continued until the end of World War II. Resumption of progress after the War began with encouragement by American medical educational missions. The Japanese medical community, as well as the nation as a whole, experienced strong cultural shock when they discovered just how far American medical science had advanced and how great a gap existed between the two countries. This stimulated a strong national desire to catch up by absorbing as much about American progress as possible. Under these circumstances, Dr. Seevers kindly offered to allow Japanese pharmacologists the opportunity to study in the Department of Pharmacology of the University of Michigan Medical School. Except for an interruption from 1971 to 1981, after Dr. Seevers retired, the Michigan fellowship program started for this purpose in 1952 has continued. To date 42 postdoctoral fellows from Japan were officially accepted into the department, not counting those who only visited for brief periods or who came outside of the formal program set up by Dr. Seevers.

Upon returning to Japan from Michigan, these fellows gradually assumed important roles in medical education and research in pharmacology. Their numbers increased to the point where they form a large group of leaders in the Japanese Pharmacological Society and are known as the "Michigan Scholars." The purpose of this report is to introduce their activities and contributions to pharmacology and related medical and pharmaceutical sciences in Japan after their return from the Department of Pharmacology at the University of Michigan Medical School. One should refer to the curriculum vitae section of this book concerning the activities of specific individuals.

I. Fellows Affiliated with Universities

Some doctors who went to Michigan already held the status of full professors in Japan (Drs. S. Hisada, T. Murano, and K. Shimamoto), but most did not. However, sooner or later many became professors and chairmen of departments (mostly pharmacology) at schools of medicine, dentistry, or pharmacy in Japan. The number of those who became professors and chairmen after returning from their Michigan experiences are 15 in medical schools and 4 each in dental and pharmacy schools. Their names are as follows:

Medical schools
Drs. T. Tanabe (Hokkaido University, 1957), E. Hosoya (Keio University, 1963), H. Ito (Yoko-

79

hama City University, 1967), K. Matsusaki (Ryukyu University, 1970), K. Nakai (Akita University, 1971), E. Hasegawa (Kyoto Prefectural Medical College, 1971), S. Takaori (Kyoto University, 1972), S. Tadokoro (Gunma University, 1972), T. Iwami (Hirosaki University, 1973), T. Furukawa (Fukuoka University, 1974), A. Sakuma (Tokyo Medical and Dental University, 1974), M. Miyasaka [Dokkyo University (psychiatry), 1974], T. Fukuda (Kagoshima University, 1977), T. Oka (Tokai University, 1974), S. Kishioka (Wakayama Medical College, 1997), and M. Yoshioka (Hokkaido University, 1998).

Dental schools
Drs. S. Iida (Hokkaido University, 1968), A. Tsujimoto (Hiroshima University, 1968), N. Katsuda (Kyushu University, 1972), and R. Inoki (Osaka University, 1978).

Pharmacy schools
Drs. S. Ueki (Kyushu University, 1966), S. Miyata (Kyoto College of Pharmacy, 1967), H. Kaneto (Nagasaki University, 1969), and M. Minami (Health Science University of Hokkaido, 1986).

Following is a list of other fellows who are or were also associated with universities as adjunct professors or as faculty members:

Medical schools
Drs. T. Akera (Keio University and Tokai University), F. Ikomi (Shinshu University), Y. Nakai (Kyoto University), I. Matsuoka (Kyoto University), T. Otani (Hokkaido University), K. Yamamoto (Shinshu University), T. Yanagita (Jikei University), T. Endo (Health Science University) and H. Togashi (Hokkaido University).

Other schools
Dr. K. Takada (Keio University, in psychology).

Some became presidents or deans of medical or other schools:

Medical schools
Drs. S. Hisada (Nagoya City University, 1969–1971), T. Murano (Wakayama Medical College, 1971–1978), K. Nakai (Akita University, 1976–1982), K. Matsusaki (Miyazaki Medical School, 1980–1986), S. Tadokoro (Gunma University, 1985–1989), T. Furukawa (Fukuoka University, 1989–1998), S. Takaori (Shimane Medical University, 1990–to date), and T. Fukuda (Kagoshima University, 1991–1993).

Other schools
Dr. A. Tsujimoto (Hiroshima University of Dentistry, 1986–1988), R. Inoki (Osaka University of Dentistry, 1989–1993), H. Kaneto (Nagasaki University of Pharmacy, 1990–1992), E. Hasegawa (Sakura City College of International Studies, 1990–to date), and S. Tadokoro (Gunma Prefectural College of Health Science, 1993–to date).

II. Fellows Affiliated with Institutions Other Than Universities

Dr. K. Yamamoto continued his research work at Shionogi Laboratories following his return from Michigan in 1965. He later became director of the Division of Neuropharmacology, then managing director of the Cell Science Research Foundation of Shionogi Laboratories.

Dr. T. Yanagita also returned from Michigan in 1965, and in the following year established a new laboratory as part of the Central Institute for Experimental Animals, a non-profit organization endorsed by the Ministry of Education of Japan. A research grant from NIMH, gained as a subcontract of Dr. Seevers' project on self-administration studies in monkeys, enabled Yanagita to establish this research facility, which was known as the Preclinical Research Laboratories. He was the director of the laboratories as well as a board member of the Institute until 1996.

Drs. N. Fukuda and K. Takada continued their research work at Takeda Chemical Industry and the Preclinical Research Laboratories, respectively, since their return from Michigan.

Several fellows joined the pharmaceutical industry following outstanding academic careers. Dr. K. Shimamoto joined Takeda Chemical Industry in 1968 and served as a top director of the research laboratories, then as a company board member. Dr. E. Hasegawa joined the Green Cross Corporation in 1978 and directed research projects as a board member. Dr. T. Murano joined Hoechst Japan in 1979 and directed research projects as a board member. Dr. T. Akera joined Merck Research Laboratories as a vice-president responsible for research projects, and subsequently moved to Banyu Pharmaceutical Company as head of R&D.

Some fellows entered into clinical fields after their academic careers and have served or are serving as directors of hospitals. They include: Dr. Y. Nakai (Nakai ENT Clinic, 1975), T. Otani (Otani Hospital, 1976), I. Matsuoka (Nagisa Hospital, 1985), F. Ikomi (Kofu City Hospital, 1985), A. Tsujimoto (Yno Hot Spring Hospital, 1991), and R. Inoki (Okanami General Hospital, 1994).

III. Activities in Pharmacological Societies in Japan

The Michigan fellows brought new concepts and methodologies into the Japanese medical and pharmaceutical communities, mainly through their activities in various pharmacological societies. The most authoritative pharmacological society in Japan is the Japanese Pharmacological Society, from which the Michigan fellows were selected and to which all Japanese pharmacologists belong. The Michigan fellows contributed im-

mensely to the progress of pharmacology through the medium of the Japanese Pharmacological Society and through other societies such as the Japanese Pharmaceutical, Biochemistry, and Physiology Societies. The fellows also made great contributions in founding new pharmacological societies since they learned from Dr. Seevers and the department about the importance of keeping up-to-date regarding the fields of clinical pharmacology, psychopharmacology, and toxicology. Thus, in 1970, Dr. Yanagita founded the Japanese Society of Clinical Pharmacology and Therapeutics with the assistance and encouragement of many Michigan fellows such as Drs. Tanabe, K. Nakai, Sakuma, and Takaori. Dr. Yanagita also founded the Japanese Society of Neuropsychopharmacology in 1971, serving as one of its three leaders who represent the fields of pharmacology, psychiatry, and psychology. Drs. Murano and Tanabe played key roles in establishing the Japanese Society of Toxicological Sciences in 1973.

Fellows who have served as secretaries of societies and have run the Societies' secretariat offices are as follows:

The Japanese Pharmacological Society
Drs. Shimamoto (1961–1968) and Takaori (1972–1990)

The Japanese Society of Toxicological Sciences
Dr. Tanabe (1973–1985)

The Japanese Society of Clinical Pharmacology and Therapeutics
Drs. Yanagita (1970–1980) and Sakuma (1980–1995)

The Japanese Society of Neuropsychopharmacology
Dr. Yanagita (1979–1995). Dr. Iida served as manager of the Research Forum of Officers in a collaborative program between industry and academia in Hokkaido.

Following is a list of those fellows who have served as presidents of societies:

The Japanese Pharmacological Society
Drs. Tanabe (1960–1961), Hisada (1965–1966), Hosoya (1970–1971), Ueki (1980–1981), Furukawa (1987–1988), Takaori (1988–1989), and Kaneto (1995–1996)

The Japanese Society of Neuropsychopharmacology
Drs. Takaori (1985–1986), Tadokoro (board chairman, 1983–1986; president, 1989–1990), Yanagita (1985–1986), Ueki (president, 1988–1989; board chairman, 1991–1993), Furukawa (1994–1995), and Fukuda (1996–1997)

The Japanese Society of Toxicological Sciences
Drs. Tanabe (1981–1982) and Yanagita (1988–1989)

The Japanese Society of Clinical Pharmacology and Therapeutics
Drs. Sakuma (1989–1990) and Yanagita (1992–1993). In addition, Dr. Miyasaka has served as president of the Japanese Societies of Epilepsy (1983–1984), Geriatric Psychiatry (1989–1990), and Psychiatry and Neurology (1992–1993). Also, to date, Dr. Minami is serving as chairman of the Hokkaido branch of the Pharmaceutical Society of Japan.

IV. Activities in International Pharmacological Societies

Many Michigan fellows have served as executive committee members or councilors in international pharmacological societies such as the International Union of Pharmacology. They have also served as hosts of international congresses in Japan. Such activities as known to the author are as follows:

Dr. Yanagita, Chairman of Program Committee, *IVth International Congress of Toxicology* (1986, Tokyo); Secretary General, *XVIIth Inter-*

national Congress of Neuropsychopharmacology (1990, Kyoto); President, *1st Conference of Asian Society of Toxicology* (1997, Yokohama).

Dr. Sakuma, Secretary General, *5th International Congress of Clinical Pharmacology and Therapeutics* (1992, Yokohama).

V. Activities in the Public Service

Many Michigan fellows were or are involved in governmental advisory committees of such bureaus as the Ministry of Education and Ministry of Health and Welfare. Many also serve as advisory board members in their communities and local government branches. Unfortunately, no reliable or complete records in this regard are available to the author, though it is known that Dr. Tanabe served for a long period as a member of the Science Council of Japan, the top council of Japanese academia.

Some fellows have served or are serving as advisory committee members of international organizations. Dr. Hosoya long served as a member of the Advisory Panel on Drug Dependence of the World Health Organization. To date, Dr. Yanagita has been serving in the same capacity since 1972. In 1994, Dr. Yanagita also served as an advisory member of the United Nations concerning the UN's drug abuse policies.

VI. Honors and Prizes

Many fellows have been honored by their universities as honorary professors following their retirement. They are (in alphabetical order): Drs. Hisada, Hosoya, Iida, Inoki, Katsuda, Matsusaki, Miyata, Murano, K. Nakai, Shimamoto, Tadokoro, Takaori, Tanabe, and Ueki.

Some fellows have also been presented awards or prizes. The names of such recipients as quoted from their curriculum vitae are: Drs. Ikomi (Kofu Mayor's Outstanding Effort Award, 1992), Furukawa (Kanae Award for Medical Research, 1972), Miyasaka (Shimazaki's Prize for Psychiatric Research, 1970), Ueki (Prize of the Pharmaceutical Society of Japan for Scientific Achievement, 1984), T. Yamamoto (Scientific Award of the Japanese Society of Neuropsychopharmacology, 1995), and Yanagita (Mochizuki Prize for Outstanding Achievement in Toxicology, 1994).

VII. Publications

A great number of studies were and are being carried out by the fellows over the past 30 years. The number of papers written is impressive. Among these publications are some outstanding books familiar to the author: Dr. H. Ito wrote *A Textbook of Pharmacology* in 1959 (one of the most popular textbooks, it was widely used by medical students especially from 1959 to the 1970s); and Dr. A. Sakuma wrote *Q & A in Medical Statistics* in 1987, which has been a very popular and long-selling book. Dr. Sakuma also translated S. Snyder's superb book *Drugs and the Brain.* Dr. Tadokoro edited *Alcohol and Drug Dependence* (1984); Dr. M. Minami edited *TDM* (1990); and Dr. Yanagita edited *Drug Dependence and Behavioral Toxicology* (1990). Drs. Sakuma, Tadokoro, and Hasegawa have written several family education books dealing with pharmacological, toxicological, or social aspects of drugs.

Section IV.   Other Japanese
Postdoctoral Research Fellows

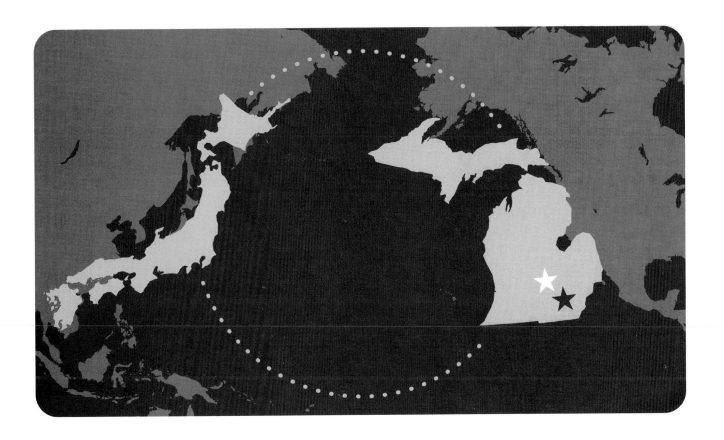

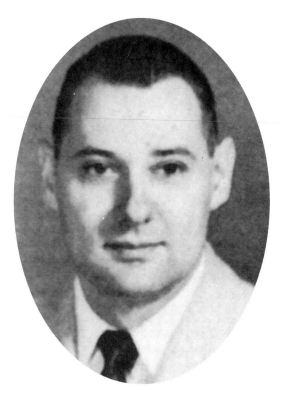

17

University of Michigan Pharmacology Japanese Research Fellows and Associates

Edward F. Domino, M.D.

As Dr. Seevers was getting older, he promoted more of the faculty of the department to full professorships. Thus, a number of us, through hard work and outside research grants, became relatively independent. Although we were all members of the same Department of Pharmacology, after he retired it became impossible to have a chairperson as strong-minded as Dr. Seevers. He taught us well. A number of us, even today, enjoy

considerable independence which weakens somewhat the strength that departmental political and scientific cooperation entails.

Dr. Seevers rapidly promoted me through the ranks. In 1954 I became an assistant professor and eight years later in 1962, I was a full professor. However, my wife, Toni, and I had five children to support, and so I needed more money than I was making in the department. Since I had a medical license to practice in both Illinois and Michigan, I was seriously considering leaving the University. In 1959, while Showa Ueki was still with me, Dr. Seevers called me into his office. Knowing my financial burdens, he asked if I would be willing to be a consultant to the Michigan Department of Mental Health, which had its best research facility, the Lafayette Clinic, in Detroit. The conditions were simple. My major job would continue to be in the Department of Pharmacology with teaching and research as priorities. I could spend one day per week plus my summer vacations working in Detroit. All grants I obtained would be through Dr. Seevers and the University of Michigan. If I could not maintain my loyalty to him and the department, he would ask me to leave. I was on a nine-month academic appointment. I was to keep in touch with Dotty Norton Overbeck regarding my ability to earn enough money to take care of my family. Finally, my number one job was to make him look good, since he was my boss.

Fig. 1. Dr. Edward F. Domino, ca. 1960.

What a wonderful arrangement! Dr. Seevers made good on all his commitments to me for the rest of his life and, in return, I got the opportunity to do both basic and clinical pharmacological research with the income that Toni and I needed to raise our family. Some years, I was on a three-ninths summer appointment for full time research as long as I could find the grant funds with which to pay myself. If I couldn't get the funds, I could also work on Seevers' projects, which included some amazing research opportunities and challenges. My consultantship at the Lafayette Clinic lasted 25 years. As a result, I never left the University of Michigan because my research and financial opportunities here in Ann Arbor were far better than any of the many chairmanships I have been offered in the United States and Canada.

With so many research opportunities, I needed graduate students, postdoctoral fellows, technicians, research associates, and assistants to work with me. This brings me especially to postdoctoral fellows from Japan. By the mid-1960s, I was being contacted directly by various M.D.s and Ph.D.s from Japan, independent of the Seevers Michigan Fellows mechanism. Dr. Seevers agreed to allow me to accept postdoctoral fellows to work in my laboratory on the condition that he could refuse to allow any fellow from Japan who he felt was inappropriate.

Dr. Hiroshi Kawamura was a key person I wished to recruit to my expanding "second" laboratory at the Lafayette Clinic. He was trained at the University of Tokyo by Professor T. Tokizane, who considered him one of his two best neurophysiologists and an expert on EEG. Hiroshi must have heard about me through Ken-ichi Yamamoto. After many negotiations, Hiroshi agreed to run my laboratory in Detroit. Though not an official Seevers fellow, he was a key person for me, and his research contributions were outstanding. For example, he showed that lesions of the pontine reticular formation blocked EEG activation of nicotine. He helped my graduate student, Jim Roppello, show that nicotine stimulates lateral geniculate neurons.

For me, there are three types of Michigan fellows. First and foremost are those who were brought to our department by Dr. Seevers, or arranged by subsequent interim, acting, and permanent chairmen (Drs. Swain, La Du, Ruddon, Counsell, and Hollenberg) if they joined the Japanese Michigan Fellows Society in Japan. After Dr. Seevers' death, the Maurice H. Seevers International Fellowship in Pharmacology was created. Those persons are the second type of Michigan fellows, of which five of the last six are Japanese. Finally, in the third group are the postdoctoral fellows who were members of our department but never joined the Society and might perhaps be forgotten. In this group, which I have listed in Table 1, are some about whom I do not know much. Hence, I am placing an emphasis on those who worked with me.

Dr. Shigeaki Matsuoka was a Japanese neurosurgeon whom I first met when I spent a summer at St. Barnabas Hospital in New York City. Dr. Seevers felt that I should do as much clinical research as appropriate, but always with a pharmacological aspect that would make our department look good. So it

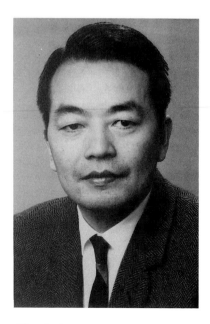

Fig. 2. A young H. Kawamura.

Table 1. Other Japanese Fellows, Dates of Stay, and the Faculty Laboratories in Which They Worked

No.	Name	Years of Stay	Mentor
1.	Shigeaki Matsuoka	1964–1965; 1967	E.F. Domino
2.	Hiroshi Kawamura	1966–1969	E.F. Domino
3.	Akie Ide	1968–1969	R.E. Counsell
4.	Koshi Hatada	1973–1974	E.F. Domino
5.	Noboyushi Iwata	1973–1974	E.F. Domino
6.	Shigetaka Naito	1979–1984	T. Ueda
7.	Hioyuke Abe	1982	R.E. Counsell
8.	Jun-ichi Shioi	1983–1985	T. Ueda
9.	Yoshiaki Wakita	1987	R.E. Counsell
10.	Yasuo Tamura	1987–1988	B.R. Lucchesi
11.	Terushi Haradahira	1988–1989	R.E. Counsell
12.	Hideo Morino	1988–1989	T. Ueda
13.	Masuru Usami	1988–1990	T. Ueda
14.	Takuzo Kishimoto	1993–1995	E.F. Domino
15.	Chitoshi Kadoya	1993–1995	E.F. Domino
16.	Taku Amano	1996–1998	T. Ueda
17.	Yutaka Tamura	1997–1998	T. Ueda

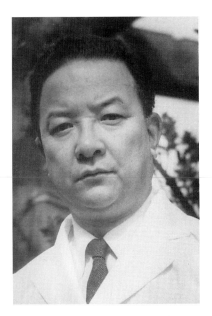

Fig. 3. Dr. Shigeaki Matsuoka while in Dr. Domino's lab.

was that I ended up in New York with all of my electronic equipment from the department, including a computer of average transients that could be used to record evoked potentials with the scalp electrodes from the EEG. The electronics were set up by Roger Lininger, who at the time was my electronics technician. Later, he ran the departmental storeroom after Bill Sheldon retired.

Dr. Irving Cooper, a famous and controversial neurosurgeon at St. Barnabas, was visiting the neurosurgery section of University Hospital, by the invitation of its head, Dr. Eddie Kahn. While there, Dr. Cooper saw me and our set-up in the anesthesia wing of University Hospital while we were studying visual evoked potentials in patients with scalp recordings, before and during general anesthesia. Dr. Guenter Corssen from the anesthesia section, and I had already shown that such scalp-recorded evoked potentials could be obtained in completely paralyzed and anesthetized surgical patients. Therefore, we knew the potentials were not skeletal artifact.

Dr. Cooper suggested I try to record such sensory evoked potentials from the sensory cortex of his patients while they underwent surgery for parkinsonism. Because of technical, ethical, and surgical considerations, the best access would be close to the primary sensory cortex. Thus, it would be possible to electrically stimulate the hand of a patient and record in the opposite brain hemisphere from both the scalp and the underlying neocortex somatosensory evoked potentials. A major neurosurgical concern was that the best cryogenic lesion at that time for parkinsonian tremors of the hand was in the contralateral ventralis lateralis (VL) near the ventralis posterior lateralis (VPL) nucleus of the thalamus. VL is the motor, but VPL is the somatosensory nucleus. Hence, too much of a lesion of VPL would cause a permanent sensory loss in the patient. Dr. Cooper wanted me to help him and his patients with that problem by coming to St. Barnabas with all of the equipment necessary, for they had none. I would be paid as a consultant for the effort.

Thus, I ended up at St. Barnabas Hospital in the Bronx, where I met Shigeaki. At the time, he had just come from the Montreal Neurological Institute, where he had worked with the famous neurosurgeon, Dr. Penfield. Shigeaki and I got along extremely well and worked together every day. Soon we were able to show in locally-anesthetized awake parkinsonian patients that somatosensory evoked potentials from the scalp are very poor, grossly attenuated responses from the underlying hand somatosensory cortex. Furthermore, if the cryogenic lesion was too large, it would dramatically alter the amplitude and shape of the evoked potential. By first simply cooling but not freezing, the reduced potential could be subsequently restored to normal by the patient's own warm blood. Wow! A theoretical and practical scientific accomplishment worthy of an article in a 1964 issue of *Science* magazine. Later, we studied the effects of cryogenic thalamic lesions on the somesthetic evoked response in both Dr. Cooper's patients in New York and in monkeys here at the University of Michigan.

Dr. S. Matsuoka stayed in Ann Arbor with his family as a postdoctoral fellow of mine.

His second of three daughters, Yayoi, and my daughter Debra were at Angell Elementary School together. When Shigeaki went back to Japan, he eventually became a professor and chairman of the Department of Neurosurgery at the University of Occupational and Environmental Health in Kitakyushu. Over the years he has told me many interesting stories, but the one I remember most is that he was a medical student in Kumamoto in August 1945, during World War II. The American plane that dropped the second atom bomb on Japan originally targeted the steelmills in Yahata, a center for chemical engineering and heavy industry. Yahata, Tobata, Wakamatsu, Kokura and Moji were combined in 1963 to form Kitakyushu currently the largest city on the island of Kyushu. The University of Occupational and Environmental Health was established in Yahata in the early 1980s and Shigeaki was appointed its first professor and chairman of neurosurgery. Clouds and haze over Yahata caused the crew of the Enola Gay, the plane carrying the atom bomb, to fly to the secondary target, Nagasaki. Years later my wife Toni and I have spent many weeks to months in Yahata at the University Guest House near the original proposed dropsite for the second atom bomb on Japan. When we both were young during World War II never could we imagine in our wildest dreams ever being there!

In 1988, Shigeaki invited me to lecture to his neurosurgical residents as a visiting professor in his department. Since then my wife and I have seen him and members of his family at least once or twice a year in Japan because of areas of mutual interest. He and Professor Shoogo Ueno, now at the University of Tokyo in the Department of Medical Electronics, developed and applied computerized brain mapping of the EEG. That methodology started both Shigeaki and me in the area of human nicotine and tobacco research, which we still continue today.

Many additional postdoctoral fellows from Japan came to Ann Arbor to work in my

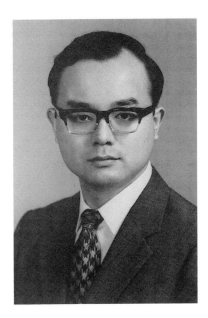

Fig. 4. Dr. N. Iwata in 1974.

laboratories. Drs. Koshi Hatada and Noboyushi Iwata were two who worked in my labs at the Lafayette Clinic in 1973-1974. They both were well-trained electrophysiologists. When they returned to Japan, Dr. Hatada went into the clinical practice of psychiatry. Dr. Iwata went to Sankyo and is now head of their neuropharmacology laboratories.

In more recent years, Dr. Chitoshi Kadoya, one of Matsuoka's young neurosurgeons, came to Michigan with his wife, Juri, to do studies in anesthesiology and neurosurgery with me and my colleagues. He did topographic brain mapping of propofol in human volunteers in anesthesia and auditory evoked potentials in epileptic patients. In his last year here, he worked in Dr. Betz's laboratory with Dr. Yang from China on a rat model of stroke.

My last Japanese postdoctoral fellow was Dr. Takuzo Kishimoto, originally from Kyoto University, where he had received an M.D. and a Ph.D. in pharmacology with Drs. Sasa and Takaori. Dr. Masashi Sasa was an associate professor in Dr. Takaori's group. Dr. Kishimoto was supported as a fellow in part by the Japanese Society of Clinical Pharmacology and partially by my own NIDA grant to study

the effects of tobacco smoking. Thus, a recent postdoctoral fellow came to our department who had been trained by Dr. Sasa and Professor Takaori. The latter was an original fellow who had been brought to the department by Dr. Seevers. When Professor Takaori retired, Dr. Sasa was offered the position of chairman and professor of pharmacology at Hiroshima University medical faculty. Since then, Dr. Sasa has invited me and my wife to Japan several times to lecture to his medical students. In Hiroshima, he introduced me to Dr. Yasuko Kohno, who is with Nippon Boehringer Ingelheim. She is a former Ph.D. student of Professor Ueki in Kyushu, and, through her company, is a supporter of the Japanese Michigan fellows. What a small world! How things come back that started in Ann Arbor with Showa Ueki and Shuji Takaori. Dr. Taku

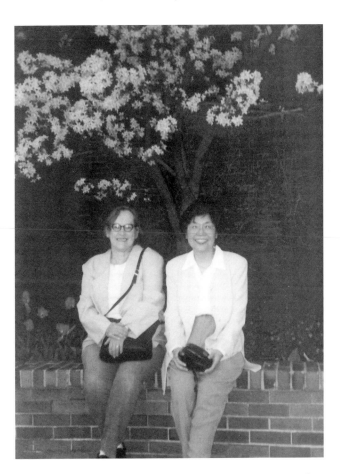

Fig. 5. Toni Domino and Dr. Y. Kohno enjoying the crabapple blossoms outside Briarwood Mall in Ann Arbor, May 1997.

Amano from Professor Sasa's group was a recent postdoctoral fellow in Dr. Tetsufumi (Ted) Ueda's laboratory at the Mental Health Research Institute and in our department.

Dr. Shigetaka Naito came to the laboratory of Dr. Ueda from the Institute for Virus Research at Kyoto University. He had a solid biochemical background and a strong desire to train in neuroscience. Dr. Ueda enormously enjoyed working and playing tennis with him. During his tenure, Dr. Naito made the following important contributions: 1) Purification of brain synaptic vesicles to morphological homogeneity, for the first time. This was achieved by using affinity-purified antibodies to synapsin I, a synaptic vesicle-specific protein. 2) Discovery of an energy-dependent, glutamate uptake system in the synaptic vesicle, suggesting that glutamate is stored within the vesicle *in vivo* in a concentrated form. 3) Basic characterization of the vesicular glutamate uptake system. This not only provided insight into the nature of the driving force of vesicular glutamate uptake, but also led to the finding that vesicular glutamate uptake is markedly stimulated by physiologically relevant low millimolar concentrations. Evidence indicated that the driving force of vesicular glutamate uptake is an electrochemical proton gradient (generated by a V-type ATPase), not a sodium gradient, which is known to serve as the driving force for cellular reuptake of glutamate. These properties, together with high affinity for glutamate, established that the vesicular glutamate uptake system is distinct from the plasma membrane glutamate uptake system. These observations allowed them to postulate that the vesicular glutamate uptake system functions as the first gate for glutamate to enter the neurotransmitter pathway, diverting glutamate away from the metabolic pathway. This gate function is of vital importance in view of the now widely accepted concept that glutamate is the major excitatory neurotransmitter in the central nervous system and, as such, plays an important role not only in basic neuronal communication but also in learning, memory, and various neurological and psychiatric disorders. Thus, his achievement in glutamate synaptic transmission represents an important contribution in neuroscience progress. After further training in Dr. Alkon's lab at NIH, Dr. Naito returned to Japan to take a research scientist position at Chugai Pharmaceutical, Inc., where he is now a laboratory director.

Dr. Jun-ichi Shioi came to Dr. Ueda's laboratory from the Dept. of Biophysics, Faculty of Science, Nagoya University. His contribution was to further elucidate the nature of the vesicular glutamate driving force. He measured the membrane potential formed by vesicular proton-pump ATPase and correlated it with vesicular glutamate uptake. He also showed that an artificially imposed membrane potential enables synaptic vesicles to take up glutamate. Dr. Shioi is now assistant professor at Mt. Sinai Medical Center School of Medicine, City University of New York.

Dr. Hideo Morino came to Dr. Ueda's laboratory from the Dept. of Neuropsychiatry, School of Medicine, Ehime University. He was concerned with glycolysis and protein phosphorylation. He purified and identified one of the phosphoproteins whose phosphorylation is stimulated by the glycolytic intermediate 3-phosphoglycerate as glucose 1,6-biphosphate synthetase. He showed that this protein was directly phosphorylated by 1,3-bisphosphoglycerate, a labile intermediate produced from 3-phosphoglycerate and ATP. He was a diligent researcher and produced solid data. He currently holds a position at Yamauchi Hospital, Ehime Prefecture.

Dr. Masaru Usami came to Dr. Ueda's laboratory from the Dept. of Internal Medicine, Kyoto University. He was engaged in studying the molecular mechanisms underlying glucose-induced insulin secretion. He found certain phosphoproteins whose phosphorylation was enhanced by phosphoglycerates. He is currently at Ikeda Hospital, Amagasaki, Hyogo Prefecture.

Dr. Taku Amano came to Dr. Ueda's laboratory from the Dept. of Pharmacology, School of Medicine, Hiroshima University. He worked on the relationship between certain forms of seizure and (a) vesicular glutamate uptake, (b) the inhibitory protein factor (IPF), a cytosolic protein which causes potent inhibition of glutamate accumulation into synaptic vesicles, and (c) synaptic proteins. He produced evidence suggesting that certain forms of seizure are associated with alterations in vesicular storage of glutamate in a specific brain region. These are strikingly interesting observations and could provide insight into the molecular mechanisms causing certain forms of seizure. Dr. Amano recently returned to Hiroshima University.

Dr. Yutaka Tamura came to Dr. Ueda's laboratory from the Dept. of Pharmacology, School of Pharmacy, Fukuyama University.

He was engaged in studies on the relationship between the regulation of vesicular glutamate uptake and exocytotically released glutamate release. He produced good evidence that the amount of exocytotically released glutamate can be varied by regulating glutamate uptake into synaptic vesicles. There had previously been no such evidence. This would open up a new avenue for investigating the modulation of glutamate transmission. He accomplished much in a short period of time. Dr. Tamura currently holds a position as lecturer at Fukuyama University.

Dr. Raymond Counsell of the department has had in his laboratory four postdoctoral fellows from Japan. All of them were truly outstanding, contributing significantly to the research effort. Dr. Akie Ide, from Ehime University, joined his staff in 1968 for one year. His two major projects were radiolabeled precur-

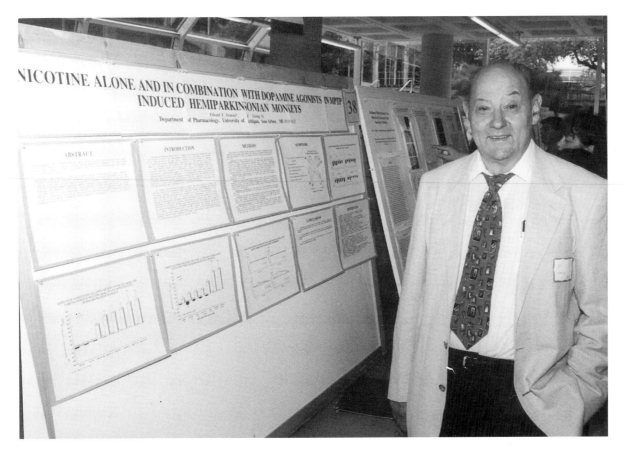

Fig. 6. An older Ed Domino still studying the effects of nicotine and his poster at a recent meeting.

sors of melanin and tyrosine hydroxylase inhibitors. His accomplishments included synthesizing both a carbon-14 labeled derivative of leucodopachrome and 3-isopropyl-*alpha*-methyl tyrosine. In 1982, after serving as a postdoctoral fellow for three years with Dr. Marino in the University of Michigan Department of Chemistry, Hioyuke Abe joined Dr. Counsell's lab for six months. During that time, he synthesized a number of adducts of testosterone as potential anti-androgens. Yoshiaki Wakita spent seven months in 1987 working with Dr. Counsell, which led to a significant amount of work and a publication. He then returned to Japan and obtained a position with the Upjohn Company in the Toxicology and Pathology division. From 1988 to 1989, Terushi Haradahira's research in Dr. Coun-

sell's lab focused on tumor-imaging agents. His work led to three publications and to the first description NM-324 which is now in clinical trials as a tumor imaging agent.

I do not have much information on others listed in Table 1, but surely each has made contributions to our Department of Pharmacology and their mentors. In the past 10 years, I have been invited to speak at many national and international meetings in Japan. Toni has been able to accompany me on almost all of these trips. As a result, we have renewed old acquaintances and made many new Japanese friends. We are privileged to have had this rare and wonderful opportunity. I only hope more persons here at Michigan will have the opportunity to mentor new postdoctoral fellows from Japan.

Michigan State University Pharmacology and Japanese Fellows

Tai Akera, M.D., Ph.D.

Fondly referred to by those at the University of Michigan as a "cow college," Michigan State University (MSU) has a world recognized College of Veterinary Medicine and is now a major multifaceted university. Pharmacology had only a minor role there prior to 1966, and was part of the physiology and pharmacology department of that college. When the College of Human Medicine was established at East Lansing in 1966, the combined Department of Physiology and Pharmacology was separated into two departments. Dr. Theodore M. Brody, then a professor in Dr. Seevers' department at the U of M, assumed the chair of the new Department of Pharmacology. He recruited several faculty members from the University of Michigan when he arrived at MSU; much of the founding faculty migrated from the U of M. This mass immigration, which continued even beyond the first years, established the relationship between the two pharmacology departments as that of a big brother and a little brother. Other than Ted Brody, who had been a professor at the U of M, graduate students Richard Rech, Kenneth Moore, David Reinke, and Gerald Gebber also eventually moved to the MSU faculty. Tai Akera, who had been a postdoctoral fellow in Dr. Brody's laboratory at the U of M from 1962 until 1964, returned to the United States from Japan in 1967 to join the MSU faculty.

After humble beginnings in the ant-infested basement of Giltner Hall, the rapidly-expanding department moved to a newly-built Life Sciences Building in 1971. While it was initially a dream building for everyone, providing ample, comfortable space, the new building also had some shortcomings. For example, in Giltner Hall one evening, a towel was accidentally left blocking the drainage of a pipette washer. The next morning, while a large area of the basement floor was found flooded, nothing had been damaged, except possibly (and hopefully) the lives of some ants. When the same accident occurred again, this time in Tai Akera's laboratory on the fourth floor of the new building, leaking water found its way into a Beckman spectrophotometer on the third floor and also damaged research papers on the second floor. The new building also could not provide for the growing department; space inadequacy proved to be such a problem that medical student laboratory courses had to be abolished in order to make more space for research.

Many of the traditions of Dr. Seevers' department at the University of Michigan were transplanted into Ted Brody's department at MSU. Fundamental to the Department of Pharmacology and Toxicology at MSU was the concept that the faculty should have a wide breadth of research interests, rather than to simply be limited to a narrow area or subdiscipline. Interests span from molecular and biochemical pharmacology to electrophysio-

Table 1. Japanese Pharmacologists Who Studied at MSU Department of Pharmacology and Toxicology

No.	Name	Years	Mentor	Current Affiliation
1.	Tai Akera	1967–1970 1971–1987	T.H. Brody	Banyu Pharmaceutical Co., Ltd.
2.	Kazuhiko Hagane	1985–1987	T. Akera	National Tochigi Hospital
3.	Tatsuya Hirota	1978–1980	G. Mayor	Koga Hospital
4.	Hiroshi Iwao	1977–1980	A. Michelakis	Osaka City Univ. Med. School
5.	Hiroyuki Izumi	1980–1982	A. Michelakis	Tohoku Univ. Sch. of Dentistry
6.	Yumi Katano	1981–1984	T. Akera	Yamagata Univ. Sch. of Medicine
7.	Keizo Maita	1981–1982	J. Hook	Inst. of Environ. Toxicology
8.	Shosei Matsumoto	1983	T. Akera	Aichi Gakuin Univ. Sch. of Dentistry
9.	Yuji Nirasawa	1983–1985	T. Akera	Kyorin Univ. Sch. of Medicine
10.	Masako Nozaki	1973–1974	T. Akera	Hokkaido Univ. Sch. of Dentistry
11.	Takeshi Okahara	1975–1976	A. Michelakis	Okahara Clinic
12.	Keisuke Takeda	1978–1980	T. Akera	Chugai Pharmaceutical Company
13.	Kyosuke Temma	1975–1977 1979–1983	T. Akera	Kitasato Univ. Sch. of Veterinary Medicine and Animal Sciences
14.	Akira Uehara	1983–1984	J. Hume	Fukuoka Univ. Sch. of Medicine
15.	Kohei Umezu	1977–1978	K. Moore	Mitsubishi Kasei Central Res. Lab.
16.	Katsushi Yamada	1981–1983	K. Moore	Kagoshima Univ. Sch. of Medicine
17.	Satoshi Yamamoto	1976–1979	T. Akera	Keio Univ. Sch. of Medicine

logical to clinical pharmacology, including cardiovascular pharmacology, neuropharmacology, smooth muscle physiology and pharmacology, behavioral and psychopharmacology, and toxicology. This diversity provides a convenient platform for pharmacologists visiting from other countries. One can always find a faculty member whose expertise and research spread into the fellow's field of interest.

Among the traditions which have carried over is a strong international flavor of the students and the postdoctoral fellows in the department at MSU. Their contributions have been essential in the success of the department. The graduates and postdoctoral fellows include individuals from Indonesia, Singapore, Hong Kong, Korea, India, and China, as well as those from Japan. During the ten-year period between 1975 and 1985, MSU hosted a large number of Japanese scholars. While many spent only one or two years in the department as postdoctoral research associates before returning to Japan, some have stayed even longer. For example, Kyosuke Temma stayed from 1975 until 1977 as a research associate, then rejoined the department in 1979 as a visiting research professor for another five years. As previously mentioned, Tai Akera had joined the MSU faculty in 1967 as a visiting assistant professor. After a brief return to Tokyo to get a permanent visa, Akera came back to MSU as an associate professor, then was later promoted to a full professor. He stayed in the United States until 1987, serving that last year after Ted Brody's retirement as acting chairman of the department.

Similarly to pharmacologists visiting Dr. Seevers' department, those arriving at the MSU campus had the benefits of an initial orientation and inheriting the essentials for surviving a Michigan winter from previous fellows. The continuous presence and turnover of these foreign scientists provided an environment where newcomers could learn from those returning to their own countries. As in Ann Arbor, used cars, used blankets, used furniture, and used anything was readily available upon arrival in East Lansing.

The weather in East Lansing is also similar to that of Ann Arbor. In the beautiful climate between May and September, visiting pharmacologists enjoy outdoor activities such as barbecuing, golfing, fishing, and tennis. MSU sports 40 outdoor tennis courts, six indoor courts, and two 18-hole golf courses. Ted Brody, a dedicated golfer, led many faculty members and visitors around those courses. Once golfers started losing balls on the putting green in piles of fallen leaves, winter could be

seen coming and the pharmacologists had to retreat back to laboratory experiments for the duration or brave the cold to take up skiing.

One aspect that distinguishes the pharmacology departments at the two universities is the tenure of the chairmanship. Following Dr. Seevers' retirement, the U of M Department of Pharmacology had a series of chairpersons, all of whom served relatively short terms. In fact, Dr. Swain was deemed to be the "permanent back-up chair," serving often as interim chairman. At MSU, Dr. Brody served as chair for 20 years (1966–1986), until he was required to retire as chairman and became a professor emeritus. After Dr. Akera served as acting chair for one year, Dr. Moore assumed the chairmanship and to date is still in that role.

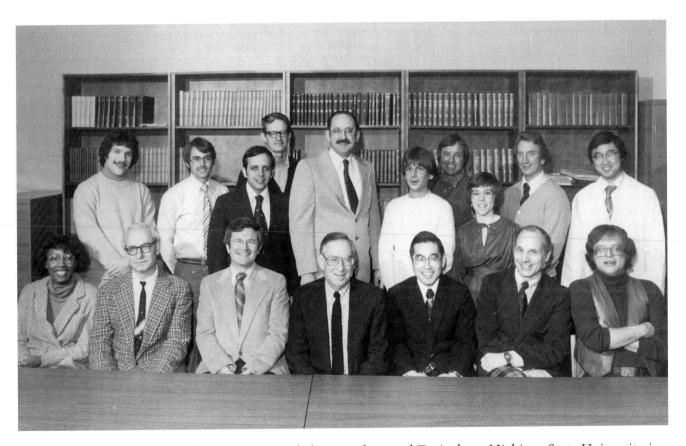

Fig. 1. Faculty members of the Department of Pharmacology and Toxicology, Michigan State University in 1978. Left to right. Front row — Janice L. Stickney, Andrew M. Michelakis, Jerry B. Hook, Theodore M. Brody, Tai Akera, Kenneth E. Moore, Gerard L. Gebber. Back row — Gregory D. Fink, Robert A. Roth, John E. Thornburg, James L. Bennett, David A. Reinke, Jay I. Goodman, Frank Welsch, Susan M. Barman, Emmett W. Braselton, Paul H. Sato.

In its early years of development, the Department of Pharmacology at MSU received a great deal of help from its "big brother." Under the leadership of Ted Brody, the Department of Pharmacology and Toxicology at MSU quickly established itself as one of the best pharmacology departments in the United States. The relationship between the two departments, however, remains excellent. Their interactions have produced important and educational results, including the Annual Graduate Student Colloquium. The brainchild of Dr. Lucchesi (at the U of M) and Dr. Rech (at MSU), this one-day event has been ongoing for many years. Begun for students at the U of M and MSU, the colloquium quickly grew to include students from Wayne State University in Detroit and the Medical College of Ohio in Toledo. Students present their research and partake in a friendly competition for recognition; judges are former faculty and students currently involved in the pharmaceutical industry.

Thirty-three years after its humble beginnings in an ant-infested basement, the Department of Pharmacology and Toxicology at Michigan State University continues to thrive and is now a first class teaching, training, and research institution thanks to Dr. Ted Brody and its current chairman, Dr. Ken Moore. The photo on the previous page is of its faculty in 1978. A positive, mature relationship exists between the two departments, and both are continuing their support of pharmacologists world-wide.

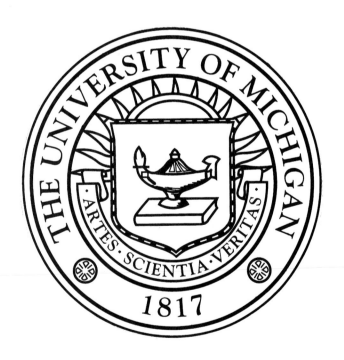

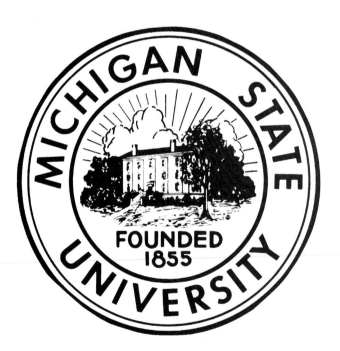

Section V.   The University of Michigan and Japan: Present and Future Collaboration

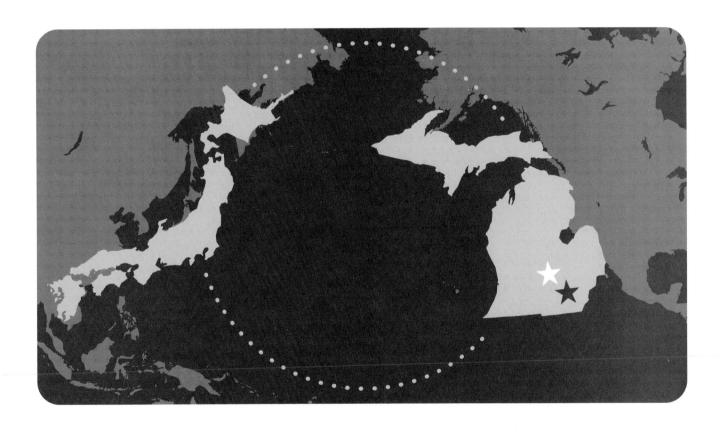

19

Reflections on our Japanese Friends

Charles B. Smith, M.D., Ph.D.

Soon after my arrival in Ann Arbor during the summer of 1966, I became aware of the established tradition of Japanese scholars visiting the Department of Pharmacology, in many instances to work in the laboratory of faculty members. It was not until the summer of 1982 that one of those scholars spent some time in our laboratory. Dr. Tsuneyuki Yamamoto was collaborating with Ellen Walker, a graduate student in the Department, on a behavioral project that involved the role of serotonin in the avian central nervous system. He came to us because he wished to measure serotonin levels in various areas of the pigeon brain and because my wife, Dr. Peggie J. Hollingsworth, who had studied cholinesterases and adrenergic receptors in the hen brain, was knowledgeable about the anatomy and neurochemistry of the avian brain. Yuki, as we called him, was bright, animated and outgoing. He brought to us his bubbling enthusiasm. Apart from the excellent research he carried out, I clearly recollect a day when a pigeon, about to face the guillotine, escaped and flew to the highest reaches of our laboratory, which in Medical Science Building I (Med. Sci. I) had extremely high ceilings. Within a flash, Yuki had nimbly clambered over benches and cabinets to capture the errant and unfortunate bird.

In addition to being a pharmacologist, Yuki was an accomplished graphic artist. When he left Ann Arbor, he gave my wife and me two of his beautiful linotype block prints, one of the Burton Memorial Tower and another of the entrance to the Rackham Graduate School during winter. Today these prints occupy a prominent position in our home. When we last met at a meeting of the Japanese Pharmacology Society in March, 1997, Yuki and I reflected on his brief sojourn in our laboratory 15 years earlier. He commented, with a characteristic twinkle in his eye, that, at heart, he still was an artist first and then a pharmacologist.

One hot summer day in 1989, two extremely proper and distinguished looking Japanese gentlemen appeared at the door of my office on the 6th floor of Med. Sci. I. This was my first encounter with Professor Hideya Saito and Dr. Mitsuhiro Yoshioka, both of whom were to become dear friends and to occupy an important place in the lives of my wife and me. Professor Saito began by thanking me profusely for agreeing to have Dr. Yoshioka spend a year in my laboratory, but he also informed me that I must return him promptly at the end of that year since Dr. Yoshioka was indispensable to Professor Saito and to the First Department of Pharmacology of Hokkaido University Medical School. At that time, I had not yet learned that it was customary for a Japanese professor to inspect the laboratory and personally evaluate the laboratory head before allowing a young faculty member to go abroad to work.

Several months later, Dr. Yoshioka, his wife, Naoka, and two young children, Yu and Dai, arrived in Ann Arbor to begin the year of his fellowship.

Dr. Yoshioka was the second Seevers International Fellow to work with us. Almost exactly a decade earlier, the first Seevers International Fellow, Dr. Jesus A. Garcia-Seville, who today heads the Department of Pharmacology at the University of the Balearic Islands, had spent two years in our laboratory. Like his predecessor, Mitsuhiro, at the time of his arrival, was already a highly productive, established pharmacologist with a sound international reputation. He worked long, hard hours, generated quantities of excellent data, and, most importantly, had a significant impact on the direction of the research that we were conducting in our laboratory. Everyone in the laboratory was most interested in learning everything possible about Japan from Mitsuhiro, and he was just as dedicated to learning as much as he could about the United States. He quickly demonstrated an unusual mastery of the English language and assimilated himself, with the single exception of the choices of the food that he ate, totally into our culture. (After having spent some time in Japan, I also tend to prefer Japanese food.) He was comfortable with the diversity of the students and staff who worked in our laboratory and went out of his way to engage himself fully in our social, as well as our work-related activities. The University of Michigan considers Martin Luther King Day to be an important occasion on our campus. At that time, it involved a week or more of events related to cultural diversity. Mitsuhiro immersed himself totally in the activities that surrounded this occasion and for months thereafter engaged us in lively and thoughtful discussions of the issues that arose during that week.

In November, 1989, Mitsuhiro, Naoka, Yu, and Dai joined other guests in our home for Thanksgiving dinner. On entering our home with a "hoop and a holler" Yu and Dai dashed down the long hallway that holds our collection of art works and literally flew into our sunken living room (something that seems quite natural for young children who come to visit our home). Later that evening, one of our guests felt compelled to instruct two year old Dai in the "proper" manner to eat his dessert. In response, and with remarkable grace and dexterity, Dai managed to propel a large spoonful of whipped cream into the face of his tormentor (much, I suspect, to the satisfaction of some of the adults present who had been more inhibited when they were that age). Several days later, we received a card from Yu and Dai with the simple message "Please forgive our bad behavior."

One day, while working in my office, the most beautiful flute music wafted into me from the laboratory. It was at that time that I learned that Mitsuhiro was a most accomplished musician who occupied the first chair in the flute section and was the musical director of the Sapporo Symphony Orchestra. He was playing his golden flute for those in the laboratory at their request. At the end of the academic year when Mitsuhiro and his family had to return to Japan, we were comforted with the knowledge that a life-long relationship had been established between us and our friends in Japan.

In June of 1991, my wife, Peggie Hollingsworth, and I made our initial trip to the First Department of Pharmacology at the Hokkaido University Medical School in Sapporo, as guests of Professor Saito and Dr. Yoshioka. Although this was not our first visit to Japan, it was the first of three of the most meaningful and wondrous visits that we were to make to that country. I will not go into detail regarding those trips since this monograph is meant to focus on the Japanese scholars who spent time in the Department of Pharmacology at the University of Michigan. During the 1991 trip, we had lunch nearly every day that we were at the University with Professor Emeritus Tsuneyoshi Tanabe, one of the early Japanese scholars to spend time at Michigan with Professor Seevers. We also re-

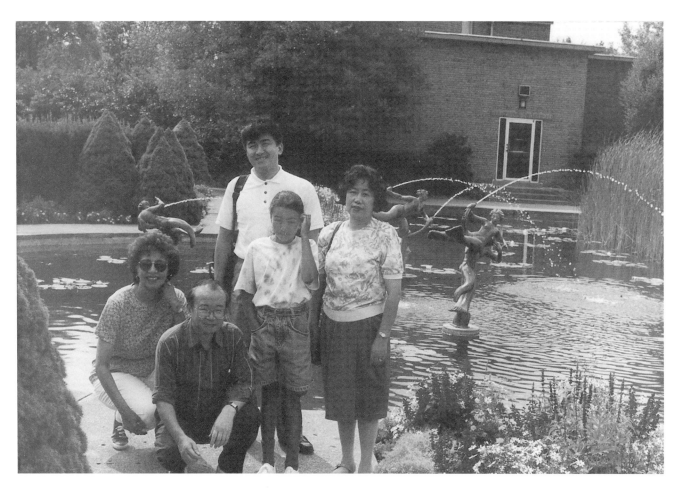

Fig. 1. Visiting Cranbrook Institute in Bloomfield Hills, Michigan, July 30, 1994. Front row from left: Dr. M. Minami, Daniela Chancy, Mrs. Minami. Back row from left: Drs. P. Hollingsworth, T. Endo.

newed our acquaintance with Professor Masaru Minami, who had worked at Michigan with Professor Lucchesi and was Professor and Chairman of the Department of Pharmacology at the Higashi-Nippon-Gakuen University. We also met Drs. Machiko Matsumoto and Hiroko Togashi, both of whom were Assistant Professors in the First Department of Pharmacology, and established an ongoing research program between our respective laboratories.

Our second trip to Sapporo was in June, 1994. At that time, Professor Minami made arrangements for Dr. Toru Endo, a young faculty member in his department, to join our laboratory group in Ann Arbor. Later that summer, as with Professor Saito and Dr. Yo-

shioka, Professor Minami and Dr. Endo visited Ann Arbor to make final arrangements in advance of the beginning of Dr. Endo's fellowship year. During that visit, Professor Minami and his wife, Dr. Endo, my wife, our nine year old granddaughter Daniela, and I took a trip to the Cranbrook Institute which houses a wonderful hands-on museum. At that time, we noted the remarkable rapport that Professor Minami had with our granddaughter as they worked through the various activities presented by that museum.

Toru spent the 1994–95 academic year in our laboratory and demonstrated the same dedication to hard work and productivity of his predecessors. He also seemed, however, to represent a generational change. He was fas-

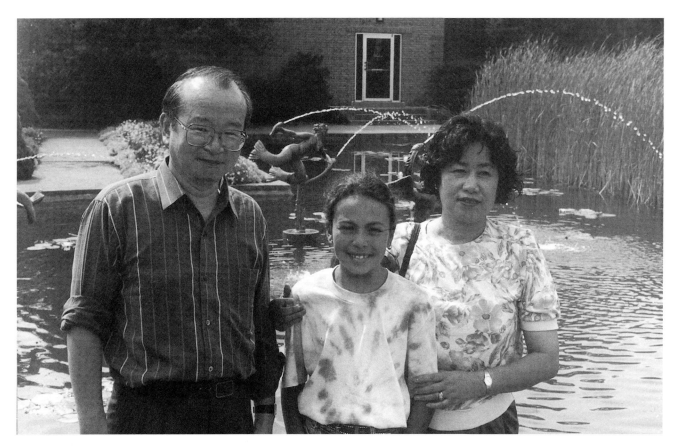

Fig. 2. Dr. and Mrs. Minami with Daniela at Cranbrook Institute, July 30, 1994.

cinated by everything American, from big cars to American food. We understood that he was an outstanding athlete and expert skier. He was gentle, kind, thoughtful and quite reserved. We thought that he would be quite a "catch" for some young lady, but at the end of his fellowship year he was still a bachelor.

During our two visits to Sapporo, we could not help but notice the exceptional qualities of two of our hosts, Drs. Matsumoto and Togashi. I tried hard to entice both of these ladies to join our laboratory in Ann Arbor but encountered resistance, which I somehow suspected emanated from Professor Saito and Dr. Yoshioka. My secret belief is they felt that, with the exception of very brief absences, the First Department of Pharmacology would not function properly without Drs. Matsumoto and Togashi. Finally, however, I did succeed in getting Dr. Hiroko Togashi to join us for several months in the summer of 1996. Upon her arrival, I immediately

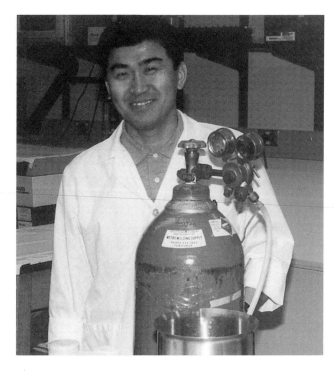

Fig. 3. Dr. T. Endo working in Dr. Smith's lab, A323 Medical Science Research Building III, November, 1994.

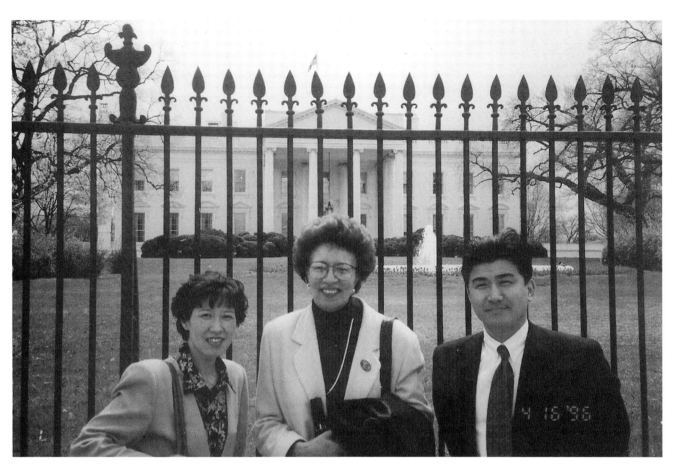

Fig. 4. Drs. H. Togashi, P. Hollingsworth and T. Endo in front of the White House, Washington, D.C., April 16, 1996.

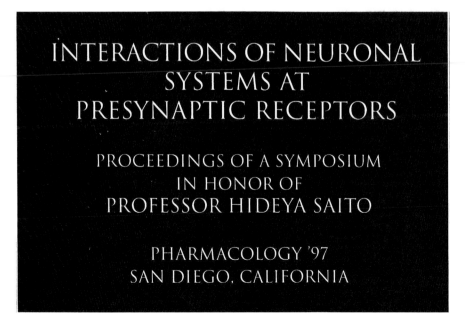

Fig. 5. Cover of the Symposium Proceedings in honor of Dr. H. Saito.

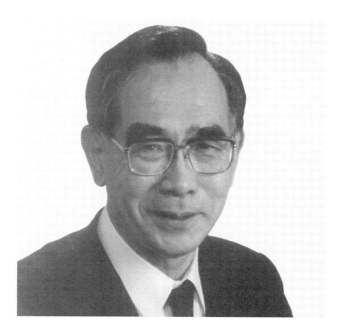

Fig. 6. Recent photograph of Dr. H. Saito.

sent an email message to Sapporo stating that now that Hiroko was in Ann Arbor, I would keep her here for at least a year. She worked hard and learned our field-stimulation techniques with remarkable rapidity. Within a few months, she generated enough data for a presentation at the next meeting of the pharmacology society. Hiroko quickly endeared herself to everyone in our laboratory. At the end of the summer when she had to return to Japan to take up her teaching duties, the young people in the laboratory cried when she departed.

I will conclude with a brief account of several events that involved our Japanese friends and colleagues during the past two years. Upon returning to Japan, Toru Endo was appointed an Assistant Professor at the Higashi-Nippon-Gakuen University in Professor Minami's department. In February, 1997, a symposium was held at the Annual Meeting of the American Society for Pharmacology and Experimental Therapeutics in honor of Professor Saito. Later in March, 1997, Professors Saito and Minami invited me to participate in a symposium at the Japanese Pharmacology Society meeting in Narita, Japan. After the meeting, Professor Saito took me and my wife on a fantastic trip to Tokyo and Kyoto, explaining that he wanted us to experience and learn first-hand about the history and culture of Japan. In May, 1997, Professor Saito retired from the First Department of Pharmacology and joined Professor Minami at Higashi-Nippon-Gakuen University. In July, 1997, the professors of the Hokkaido University Medical School elected Mitsuhiro Yoshioka Professor and Chairman of the First Department of Pharmacology. My hope is that the ties established between our friends and colleagues in Japan and us will last forever.

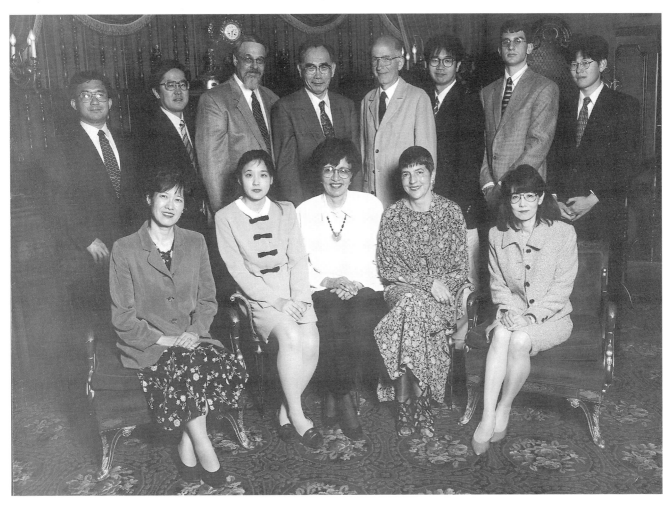

Fig. 7. Guests at the banquet in honor of Dr. H. Saito at Mr. A's Restaurant, San Diego, California, March 10, 1997.
Front row from left: Drs. H. Togashi, Kumi Saito, P. Hollingsworth, Mrs. M. Starke, Dr. M. Matsumoto.
Back row from left: Drs. K. Miyata, M. Yoshioka, C.B. Smith, H. Saito, K. Starke, Katsuhara Saito, Mr. J.D. Smithers, Dr. K. Mori.

20

Recent Experience With a Japanese Fellow and My Trip to Japan

Margaret E. Gnegy, Ph.D.

In 1993, I had a fortunate experience. I was contacted by a Japanese scientist, Dr. Shin-ichi Iwata, who wished work in my laboratory to develop his interest in dopamine. Dr. Iwata was a recipient of a Maurice Seevers Postdoctoral Fellowship and spent from June, 1994 to June, 1996 in my laboratory. He was highly intelligent, industrious and a most pleasant person. Everyone in the laboratory soon became attached to Shin-ichi, his charming wife, Mikayo, and his darling young son, Tomoyuki. They also enjoyed America, visiting such places as Orlando, Florida, the Yellowstone and Grand Teton National Parks in Wyoming, and Birch Run, Michigan. The latter has a large shopping center and was most enjoyed by Mikayo.

The years that Shin-ichi spent in my laboratory were scientifically highly productive. His project was to determine if two calmodulin binding proteins in rat striatum, neuromodulin and synapsin I, were phosphorylated at specific sites as a result of repeated amphetamine treatment. Both of these proteins, as well as calmodulin, have been implicated in neurotransmitter release. After repeated amphetamine, using a regimen that leads to behavioral sensitization, there is an enhanced stimulus-induced release of dopamine in rat striatum compared to controls. Using state-specific antibodies, Shin-ichi demonstrated that the phosphorylation of neuromodulin at serine-41, its protein kinase

C substrate site, and the phosphorylation of synapsin I at site 3, its calmodulin-dependent protein kinase II substrate site, were enhanced as a result of repeated amphetamine. He found that the increased phosphorylation was persistent and developed with time following cessation of drug. In a most interesting experiment, he found that incubation of synaptosomes from rats receiving repeated amphetamine also exhibited enhanced phosphorylation, suggesting that an altered enzyme activity was involved. These experiments further supported the contention that repeated amphetamine elicits a state of plasticity resembling other 'learning' models such as long term potentiation. In a final and novel series of experiments, Shin-ichi demonstrated that incubation of synaptosomes from naive rats with amphetamine could elicit the phosphorylation of neuromodulin and synapsin I at those specific sites. Therefore, amphetamine does something to induce a phosphorylation of these proteins *in vitro*. This opened up a new line of research in my laboratory in which we found that the 'reverse transport' of dopamine through the plasmalemmal transporter required protein kinase C activity. Shin-ichi wrote three first author papers while in my laboratory, two were published in the Journal of Pharmacology and Experimental Therapeutics and one in Synapse.

A highly exciting consequence of having Shin-ichi in my laboratory was that I was in-

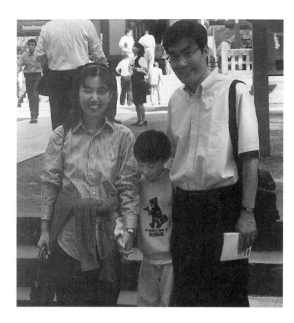

Fig. 1. Mikayo, Tomoyuki and Shin-ichi Iwata, 1997.

vited by Dr. T. Fukuda, Shin-ichi's Professor of Pharmacology in Kagoshima, to come to Japan to give two lectures in October, 1997. It was a great honor for me. My husband, Wes, accompanied me to Japan. We both love traveling abroad and absorbing different cultures. We were met at the airport in Kagoshima by Shin-ichi, Mikayo, and Tomoyuki. They de-

lighted us by taking us to a Japanese Inn in the countryside near Kagoshima and treating us to a fabulous feast of Japanese food. I think they were a bit surprised at how Wes and I enjoyed Japanese food and Japanese culture. We didn't always know what we were eating but it all tasted wonderful and we ate as much as we possibly could. We very much enjoyed the traditional inn and even partook of the public baths.

After another day of sightseeing, the meetings began. The first was an international meeting on dopamine with a marvelous roster of speakers and I found it most interesting. I was honored to meet Dr. T. Fukuda and Dr. T. Yanagita, who organized the meeting with many Japanese scientists who had studied at the University of Michigan. In the meantime, my husband had spent the warm fall day touring Kagoshima on foot. That night we had a most sumptuous banquet and I met many distinguished Japanese scientists.

An incident the next day disrupted my concentration during my second lecture which was part of the annual meeting of the Society of Neuropsychopharmacology. It

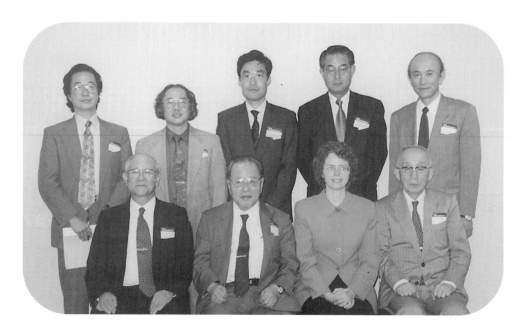

Fig. 2. Japanese pharmacologists with Dr. Gnegy during the Society of Neuropsychopharmacology meeting in Kagoshima in October, 1997.

served to underscore to us the kindness and graciousness of the Japanese people. In the morning, Wes was gripped with a terrible pain and could barely move. I found Shin-ichi who enlisted help in taking Wes to the hospital. I stayed to give my lecture which was primarily on Shin-ichi's work in my laboratory. Wes was diagnosed as having a kidney stone, probably from increased salt in the diet with insufficient water intake. Shin-ichi arranged everything at the hospital including the ultrasound and necessary medicine. Wes was able to come back to the hotel and recover there. Both Shin-ichi and Dr. Fukuda were wonderfully helpful. Dr. Fukuda graciously allowed us to stay an extra day in the hotel until Wes recovered and was solicitous concerning our needs. The hospital bill was so reasonable, compared to American prices, that we thought it might be cheaper to fly to Japan to be treated for a kidney stone than to stay at home. Wes recovered very nicely and we spent our next few days in Kyoto, a gorgeous city that reminded me of Paris.

I cannot expound enough on the friendliness and helpfulness of the Japanese people. This includes Tetsufumi (Ted) and Yasuko Ueda at the University of Michigan, who were helpful in educating us before we went to Japan. Everyone I met was gracious and kind. The country was beautiful and the food delicious. My husband and I have very fond memories of our journey. So having Dr. Shin-ichi Iwata in my laboratory was rewarding not only scientifically but also culturally in that I learned much more about a wonderful country and its gracious people.

21

University of Michigan Pharmacology Today, Including Current Research Activities

William B. Pratt, M.D.

The University of Michigan is one of the world's major research universities, and it is one of only two public institutions consistently ranked among the top 10 universities in the United States. Consisting of 17 schools and colleges, the University of Michigan's Ann Arbor campus serves 35,000 students, of which 15,000 are graduate and professional students. In the sciences, Michigan has a wide variety of graduate programs and is number one in the United States in sponsored research funding. The availability of virtually any research technology, one of the five largest library systems in the United States, and one of the largest concentrations of computers of any campus or corporation attracts scientists from all over the world to Ann Arbor to develop their ideas.

The Department of Pharmacology is located in a new research building within the medical campus, which is immediately adjacent to the University of Michigan's central campus. The medical campus contains the University Hospital, and the Schools of Medicine, Nursing and Public Health, and is home for more than 15 graduate programs in the biomedical sciences. Within this complex, the Department of Pharmacology occupies three floors of Medical Science Research Building III, with other laboratories being located in the adjacent buildings housing the Upjohn Center for Clinical Pharmacology and the Mental Health Research Institute. The major pro-

grams of the department in neuropharmacology, signal transduction, addiction research, cardiovascular pharmacology, cancer pharmacology, drug metabolism and pharmacogenetics have established the reputation of the University of Michigan as a leading international center for research and training in pharmacology.

I. Early History

The University of Michigan, founded in 1817, has a long and distinguished history. By the end of the 19th century, the University of Michigan was the largest and most generously supported public university in America and a leader in the field of graduate education. Indeed, the University has awarded more doctoral degrees than any other institution in North America.

In 1891, the University established the first Department of Pharmacology in North America, and over the more than 100 years since, it has awarded the largest number of Ph.D.s in the discipline. These graduates have made a major impact on the field of pharmacology, and they currently include many pharmaceutical company executives, research directors and senior scientists, directors of government research laboratories and leaders in academia. The scientific output of its faculty and students and the accomplishments of its graduates have served to maintain the department's position as one of the most highly regarded departments in the world.

II. Ann Arbor Today

Ann Arbor, with a population of 109,000, of whom about 36,000 are students, is located in an area of southeastern Michigan known for its lakes and scenic state parks. The University plays a major role in attracting people from all over the world to live in the city. This diversity of perspective contributes to the city's reputation as a major educational and cultural center. Ann Arbor is a pleasant place to live, with a small downtown containing about 170 restaurants and outdoor cafés with all varieties of ethnic cuisine, 83 parks, nature preserves and recreational areas, beautiful tree-lined streets and an extensive system of bike paths. Along with Cambridge, Massachusetts, Madison, Wisconsin, and Berkeley, California, Ann Arbor is considered one of the four major university cities in the United States. With its four musical series, its renowned School of Music, the largest art fair in the country, professional and student theater, opera, and dance productions, it is not surprising that the University of Michigan has been named the premier cultural environment among all American campuses.

III. The Department Today

Today, the Department of Pharmacology has 25 full-time faculty, of whom 12 maintain joint appointments in other departments or programs within the Medical School or in other schools, such as the Schools of Public Health, and Dentistry. Although the department faculty teaches several basic courses administered to more than 600 students annually, we are a research department and the great majority of faculty time is devoted to research. The department has modern facilities and equipment for performing all of the routine procedures of molecular biology, bio-

chemistry, and both cellular and organ system physiology. The Taubman Medical Library and core facilities for electron microscopy, confocal imaging studies, nucleic acid synthesis, and peptide sequencing and synthesis are immediately adjacent to the department offices. Core facilities for the production of transgenic and gene "knockout" animals are also readily available. I have included here a brief description of the research currently being conducted in the laboratories of the faculty of the Department of Pharmacology.

Signal Transduction/Neuropharmacology
(Drs. Domino, Fisher, Gnegy, Holz, Isom, Medzihradsky, Neubig, Shayman, Smith, Ueda and Woods)

One of the department's largest areas of graduate training is in neuropharmacology. Several of the laboratories in this area are working on the fundamental mechanisms by which neurotransmitter binding to receptors is transduced into the molecular events that determine the cell response. At the receptor level, Dr. Isom utilizes the techniques of molecular biology to study the functional domains of voltage-sensitive sodium ion channels and Dr. Medzihradsky focuses on the way in which the lipid environment of the cell membrane affects the conformation of drug binding sites on opioid receptors. Dr. Neubig's laboratory studies receptor-mediated signal transduction via the G protein transducers, using peptides derived from receptor sequences to determine specific sites of receptor-G protein interaction. Fluorescence spectroscopic and rapid kinetic methods are used to study the conformational changes that accompany signaling.

Receptor-mediated inositol lipid breakdown by phospholipase C occurs throughout the nervous system and leads to the production of the second messengers inositol trisphosphate and diacylglycerol with subsequent linkage to calcium signaling and protein phosphorylation. Dr. Fisher's laboratory studies the way in which receptors coupled to

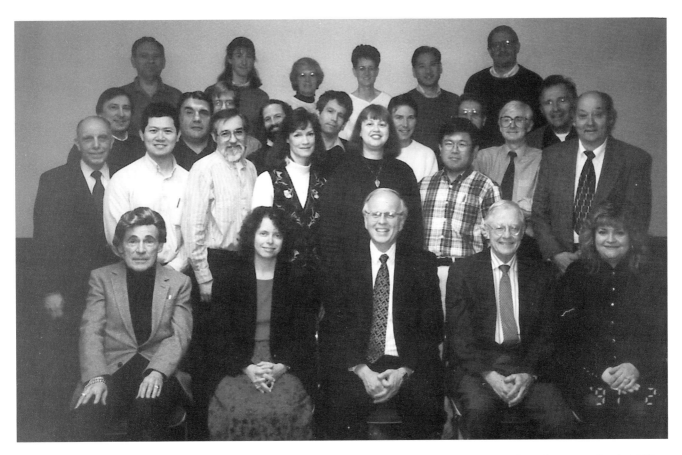

Fig. 1. Teaching and Research Faculty, Department of Pharmacology, University of Michigan, Feb. 6, 1997.

phospholipase C are internalized and how inositol lipid availability and inositol phosphate production are regulated. Dr. Shayman's laboratory is concerned with lipid signaling. Much of the role of calcium in transducing signals is determined by the calcium-binding protein calmodulin. Dr. Gnegy's laboratory focuses on muscarinic receptor regulation of calmodulin binding to calmodulin-binding proteins in neuroblastomas and the role of dopamine in the phosphorylation of calmodulin-binding proteins, such as synapsin I, in the brains of amphetamine-sensitized animals.

Drs. Holz and Ueda carry out fundamental studies on the process of neurotransmitter secretion from vesicles. Dr. Holz's laboratory uses biochemical and molecular genetic techniques to study the effects of specific proteins on regulated exocytosis in adrenal chromaffin cells and other model systems. Dr. Ueda's laboratory studies the neurotransmitter vesicles

of the synapse with special focus on how glutamate uptake into and release from brain synaptic vesicles is regulated and the role of protein phosphorylation in synaptic vesicle function.

Three laboratories in the neuropharmacology area are studying the effects of drug administration to animals on brain function and behavior. Dr. Smith's laboratory has been evaluating the way disease states, such as affective and anxiety disorders, as well as the administration of a variety of psychoactive drugs are related to abnormalities of synaptic transmission. Using quantitative EEG, evoked potential and PET techniques, Dr. Domino's laboratory is concerned with the way in which brain function is altered by psychoactive drugs including nicotine and tobacco smoking. Dr. Woods' laboratory focuses on the relationship between drug binding to receptors and the behavioral effects of the drugs using a variety of unconditioned and conditioned behaviors in birds, rodents and primates.

Drug Distribution and Metabolism and Regulation of Gene Expression
(Drs. Brenner, Counsell, Domino, Harris, Hollenberg, Osawa, Piper, Simpson, Somerman, Watkins and Weber)

The study of drug metabolism is a major area of emphasis in the department. Dr. Hollenberg's laboratory studies the microsomal P450-dependent mixed-function oxidases, which are responsible for metabolic activation and/or detoxication of many drugs, toxins and xenobiotics. Using several forms of purified P450 in a reconstituted system consisting of NADPH-P450 reductase, phospholipid and cytochrome P450, the Hollenberg laboratory studies the mechanisms of oxygen activation and substrate oxygenation and the way in which other components of the endoplasmic reticulum affect the catalytic activity of P450. Mechanism-based inactivators are being used to investigate the structures of the active sites of P450. Dr. Osawa is studying the mechanisms by which free radicals, such as nitric oxide and superoxide, interact with cellular targets and the regulation of oxidative enzymes, such as nitric oxide synthase and prostaglandin synthase, that are responsible for generation of these reactive intermediates. Dr. Watkins is interested in phenotyping all of the major families of P450s in humans and is the Director of the General Clinical Research Center in University Hospital. Dr. Domino is interested in phenotyping and genotyping CYP2A6.

Dr. Piper and Dr. Harris are toxicologists with interests in drug metabolism and protection from oxidant injury. Dr. Piper studies the way in which heme synthesis and catabolism controls the expression of hemoproteins and how hypothalamic and pituitary peptide hormones regulate cytochrome P450-mediated reactions in the biosynthesis of steroid hormones. Dr. Harris uses rodent whole embryo culture systems and conceptual primary cell cultures to study the mechanisms of embryotoxicity and the genesis of birth defects. His laboratory studies the way in which glutathione and related antioxidant enzymes protect the embryo from chemical toxicants and changes in the embryonic environment.

Drs. Brenner and Counsell are interested in drug kinetics and disposition. Using a rabbit model he has developed to study pharmacokinetics in normal and in hepatic or renal disease states, Dr. Brenner evaluates the resulting changes in drug metabolism and toxicity. Dr. Counsell's laboratory evaluates various strategies for site-specific delivery of drugs. Targeting via receptor-mediated endocytosis is a specific area of interest.

Two laboratories utilize the techniques of molecular biology to study how hormones and differentiation factors regulate gene expression. Operating through nuclear receptors the calciotropic hormone 1,25 dihydroxyvitamin D_3 regulates the growth and maturation of a variety of cell types. Dr. Simpson's laboratory has shown that 1,25 dihydroxyvitamin D_3 controls the transcription of genes for several protein kinase C isoenzymes. His research is directed at identifying both the transcriptional regulation factors and the protein kinase C substrates involved in signal transduction by the hormone. Dr. Somerman is studying the roles of two adhesion molecules, bone sialoprotein and osteopontin, in bone and connective tissue development, maintenance and regeneration. The influence of protein kinase isoenzymes on osteopontin gene expression is one focus of the work and a second series of studies is directed at determining whether the mineralization-specific bone sialoprotein is critical to the mineralization process itself.

It is now known that there are hundreds of genetic differences in human subpopulations determining drug responses that are different from the majority of individuals. The study of these genetic polymorphisms constitutes a basic subfield of pharmacology called pharmacogenetics. Dr. Weber's laboratory studies genetically polymorphic drug acetylation enzymes in both humans and animal models, using the techniques of molecular biology, which now permit rapid screening of human genes for mutations in enzymes involved in drug activation and metabolism.

Cancer Pharmacology
(Drs. Brenner, Counsell, Ensminger, Hollenberg, Mancini, Maybaum, Pratt, Shewach and Simpson)

The Cancer Pharmacology Program at the University of Michigan is comprised of a broad spectrum of investigators from the Department of Pharmacology, the College of Pharmacy, and clinical departments in the Medical School. It focuses on developing experimental approaches to the clinical treatment of cancer through research that bridges the fields of molecular carcinogenesis, biochemical pharmacology, radiation biology and clinical pharmacology. The mechanistic concepts developed in cultured cells are examined in animal models and then taken to clinical trials.

Drs. Counsell and Ensminger focus on the delivery and disposition of anticancer drugs. Because of the anatomy of hepatic blood flow and the relatively high intrinsic tolerance of normal liver cells to several anticancer drugs, tumors in the liver can be treated by pumping drugs directly into that organ through a cannula implanted in the hepatic artery. Dr. Ensminger is an expert in this form of regional drug delivery and combines this approach with gene therapy and activation of drugs by ultrasound to develop new combined modality therapies for treatment of cancers restricted to specific regions that, like the liver, can be exposed selectively to drugs. Dr. Counsell's laboratory develops compounds that are specifically designed to be retained in tumors versus normal cells. When appropriately radiolabeled, the retention of the compounds by the tumor allows visualization by whole body gamma scanning.

Two major interests of investigators in the Cancer Pharmacology Program are the study of cell killing by nucleoside analogs and the enhancement of cell killing by X-irradiation. The nucleoside analogs require activation within the cancer cell by phosphorylation to nucleotides that then interfere with DNA synthesis to cause cell death. Dr. Shewach develops methods of enhancing drug activation, both by biochemical manipulation of existing enzymes in the activation pathway and by using gene transfer techniques to express enzymes not normally present in humans but which are superior activators of the nucleoside analogs. Such gene transfer techniques can be used in cultured cells to overcome drug resistance, an approach that is being used by several investigators in the program. Dr. Maybaum is interested in the mechanisms by which nucleoside analogs and some other anticancer drugs initiate the process of apoptosis, or programmed cell death. Although the biochemical pathways of drug damage are often very well defined, the damage itself triggers the expression of genes that initiate and carry out the death process and these events are being probed with the tools of molecular biology. Dr. Mancini studies the biochemical mechanisms of sensitivity and resistance to DNA damaging agents. Novel nucleoside analogs are being investigated in cultured human leukemia cells and chemosensitizing compounds are being evaluated in malignant glioma cells in culture as a means to treat tumors that are resistant to anticancer drugs that act via DNA alkylation.

Studies on carcinogenesis are being carried out by Drs. Hollenberg and Brenner. Dr. Hollenberg is developing specific inactivators of different forms of P450 that activate carcinogens, the ultimate goal being to protect subpopulations exposed to specific carcinogens from developing cancer. P450 enzymes play a critical role in the activation and detoxication of the nitrosamine carcinogens, which are of great concern because of widespread human exposure. Dr. Hollenberg's laboratory is studying the P450s responsible for nitrosamine activation, the effects of inducing agents on their expression, and the effect of chemoprotective antioxidants on cytochrome P450 levels and carcinogen metabolism. Dr. Domino's laboratory is studying the phenotyping and genotyping of CYP2A6 and relationship to the tobacco derived nitrosamine NNK. Dr. Brenner conducts both laboratory and clinical studies aimed at lowering the incidence of carcinogenesis in susceptible populations by the long-term administration of chemopreventive agents.

Certain carcinogens (e.g., dioxin), anticancer drugs (e.g., glucocorticoids) and differentiation promoting agents (e.g., vitamin D_3) act through nuclear receptors that regulate gene expression. To be functional, the receptors for dioxin and glucocorticoids must be properly folded by heat shock protein chaperones and then must travel through the cytoplasmic and nuclear space to occupy a few copies of regulatory sequence within the genome. Dr. Pratt's laboratory studies this mechanism of protein folding and the relationship between the folding system and subsequent targeted protein trafficking through the cellular space. Dr. Simpson's laboratory studies the mechanism by which 1,25 dihydroxyvitamin D_3 promotes cell differentiation *in vitro,* with the ultimate goal of using differentiation promoters as a means of cancer treatment.

The Cancer Pharmacology Program is part of The University of Michigan Cancer Center, which is one of 25 national centers for research on and treatment of cancer. The Cancer Center includes the new cancer hospital adjacent to the basic science laboratories, the NIH-funded Cancer Biology Training Program, which funds several pharmacology graduate students, and over 100 different laboratories which reflect a broad range of expertise and interest. Most Pharmacology Department faculty who are in the Cancer Pharmacology Program have laboratories located in the Upjohn Center for Clinical Pharmacology, which is located in the center of the medical building complex.

Cardiovascular Pharmacology
(Drs. Counsell, Holz, Lucchesi, Neubig, Osawa, Shlafer and Simpson)

Cardiovascular disease is the major cause of death in the United States. The development of a basic understanding of the pathophysiology of cardiovascular disease and the development of new drugs and their preclinical testing has been a long-term focus of the Department of Pharmacology.

Dr. Lucchesi's laboratory is a major training site for students, postdoctoral fellows and clinician scientists. This large and highly regarded laboratory is supported by the longest continually- funded grant of the Heart, Lung and Blood Institute, as well as by other grants from the NIH, support from the American Heart Association and collaborations with pharmaceutical manufacturers. One major area of interest is to identify, characterize, and evaluate drugs that prevent ventricular fibrillation, the most lethal of all cardiac rhythm disturbances. A person suffering from a heart attack suffers myocardial damage, both during the ischemic phase when blood flow to regions of the heart is diminished or absent, and during the reperfusion phase when blood flow is increased again as a result of drug treatment and/or angioplasty. Dr. Lucchesi's laboratory has developed models for analyzing the pathophysiological basis for myocardial injury and the pharmacological protection of the ischemic heart. Current approaches of interest focus on the induction of the myocardial stress proteins (so-called heat shock proteins) and the analysis of how the endogenous stress response can be utilized for therapeutic protection of the heart. Major pathophysiological studies focus on the role of the immune system in causing myocardial damage, for example through leukocyte-derived oxygen free radicals and through complement mediated membrane damage. In that a heart attack usually results from coronary artery thrombosis resulting from platelet aggregation and platelet interaction with the vascular endothelium, a third focus of the laboratory is on the pharmacological control of the coronary circulation through drugs that prevent thrombosis.

Drs. Osawa and Shlafer are interested in the effects of active radical forms of oxygen on cells and tissues. Free radicals, such as nitric oxide and superoxide, and other chemically reactive compounds play important roles in a variety of pathological and physiological processes, including myocardial ischemia and reperfusion injury. The major interest of Dr. Shlafer's laboratory is to identify sources of cytotoxic oxygen metabolites generated by the heart tissue itself, their pathways of formation, and the targets they attack. Also important is the definition of endogenous defenses against oxygen metabolites and the development of methods of protecting the heart from injury during ischemia, reperfusion, or both. Dr. Osawa's laboratory focuses on the effects of free radicals on biological systems at the molecular level, again with the focus on developing rational treatments of conditions due to inappropriate free radical formation.

The medulla of the adrenal gland secretes adrenalin and other substances that increase blood pressure and control other responses of the cardiovascular system. Dr. Holz studies the fundamental process by which these vasoactive compounds are secreted from adrenal cells. One of the types of receptors that controls blood pressure is the α_2 class of adrenergic receptors, and Dr. Neubig investigates the coupling of α_2 receptors to the G-protein effectors that mediate responses.

Dr. Counsell has a long-standing interest in atherosclerosis. He has synthesized a number of radioiodinated cholesterol derivatives that have proven useful in imaging tissue cholesterol deposits using gamma camera scintography. In collaboration with Dr. Newton, Dr. Counsell's laboratory has labeled the core components of lipoproteins, such as low density lipoproteins (LDL), with various radioiodinated cholesterol probes. These radiolabeled lipoproteins are used to study choles-

terol uptake and storage and to monitor the effects of lipid-lowering drugs.

Dr. Simpson was the first to demonstrate direct effects of vitamin D_3 in regulating cardiovascular function. At the cellular level, he now studies the effect of vitamin D_3 in promoting the differentiation of cardiac myocytes in culture. These studies utilize molecular biological probes to monitor hormone-induced changes in myocyte gene expression.

Through the efforts of these faculty, their students and collaborators, the department is making important contributions to both the fundamental understanding of problems associated with cardiovascular disease and the development of new therapies.

Addiction Research
(Drs. Domino, Medzihradsky, Smith, and Woods)

Several faculty members in the department have a long-standing interest in the pharmacology of opioids and other substances with abuse liability. For more than 25 years, these investigators have made major contributions to the study of the abuse of investigational compounds with analgesic properties. Compounds from a wide variety of sources (e.g., the World Health Organization, the National Institute on Drug Abuse, and academic chemists) are assessed through this program, and the findings have led to the introduction of new analgesics with reduced human abuse liability and to the identification of abuse liability of potential new therapeutics. Through both teaching and research, the faculty also contribute significantly to a University-wide Center on Substance Abuse. A large number of students from many countries, both graduate and postdoctoral, have received addiction research training in the department.

The faculty are interested in the basic mechanisms by which opioids exert their biological and behavioral actions. Dr. Medzihradsky studies the signal transduction pathways for different opioid receptors, and Dr.

Smith studies the actions of opioids and related compounds on receptors present in smooth muscle. Dr. Woods investigates opioid actions in a variety of physiological and behavioral preparations in rhesus monkeys, including procedures that involve opioid drug-taking.

The faculty are also interested in other substances of abuse. Phencyclidine and related substances have been discovered to work through excitatory amino acid receptors, and Drs. Domino and Woods have performed extensive research on these compounds at the molecular, physiological, and behavioral levels. It is likely that new therapeutic agents for neurological disorders will be derived from this class of pharmacological agents. In addition, Dr. Domino also studies the actions of nicotine and tobacco smoking in humans and animals.

IV. Faculty of the Graduate Program in Pharmacology

Dean E. Brenner, M.D. — Hahnemann Medical College, *Professor of Internal Medicine and Associate Professor of Pharmacology*

Edward F. Domino, M.D. — University of Illinois, *Professor of Pharmacology*

William D. Ensminger, M.D. — Harvard University; Ph.D. — Rockefeller University, *Professor of Pharmacology and Professor of Internal Medicine*

Stephen K. Fisher, Ph.D. — Birmingham University (England), *Associate Professor of Pharmacology and Research Scientist, Mental Health Research Institute*

Margaret E. Gnegy, Ph.D. — University of West Virginia, *Professor of Pharmacology*

Craig Harris, Ph.D. — University of North Carolina, Chapel Hill, *Associate Professor of Toxicology, Department of Environmental and Industrial Health, School of Public Health, and Assistant Professor of Pharmacology*

Paul F. Hollenberg, Ph.D. — University of Michigan, *Maurice H. Seevers Collegiate Professor and Chair of Pharmacology*

Ronald W. Holz, M.D., Ph.D. — Albert Einstein Medical School, *Professor of Pharmacology*

Lori L. Isom, Ph.D. — Vanderbilt University, *Assistant Professor of Pharmacology*

Benedict R. Lucchesi, M.D., Ph.D. — University of Michigan, *Professor of Pharmacology*

William R. Mancini, Ph.D. — State University of New York at Buffalo, *Assistant Professor of Pharmacology*

Jonathan Maybaum, Ph.D. — University of California, San Francisco, *Professor of Pharmacology and Associate Professor of Radiation Oncology*

Richard R. Neubig, M.D., Ph.D. — Harvard University, *Professor of Pharmacology and Associate Professor of Internal Medicine*

Yoichi Osawa, Ph.D. — University of Michigan, *Assistant Professor of Pharmacology*

Walter N. Piper, Ph.D. — Purdue University, *Professor of Toxicology, Department of Environmental and Industrial Health, School of Public Health and Professor of Pharmacology*

William B. Pratt, M.D. — Yale University, *Professor of Pharmacology*

James A. Shayman, M.D. — Washington University, *Professor of Pharmacology and Professor of Internal Medicine*

Donna S. Shewach, Ph.D. — University of Texas, *Associate Professor of Pharmacology*

Marshal Shlafer, Ph.D. — Medical College of Georgia, *Professor of Pharmacology*

Robert U. Simpson, Ph.D. — University of Wisconsin, Madison, *Professor of Pharmacology*

Charles B. Smith, M.D., Ph.D. — Harvard University, *Professor of Pharmacology*

Martha J. Somerman, D.D.S. — New York University, Ph.D. — University of Rochester, *Professor of Dentistry, and Chair, Department of Periodontics/ Prevention and Geriatrics, School of Dentistry and Professor of Pharmacology, Medical School*

Tetsufumi Ueda, Ph.D. — University of Michigan, *Professor of Pharmacology, Department of Psychiatry, Professor of Pharma-*

cology and Research Scientist, Mental Health Research Institute

Paul B. Watkins, M.D. — Cornell University, *Professor of Pharmacology and Professor of Internal Medicine*

James H. Woods, Ph.D. — University of Virginia, *Professor of Pharmacology and Professor of Psychology*

Emeritus Faculty

Raymond E. Counsell, Ph.D. — University of Minnesota, *Active Emeritus Professor of Pharmacology and Professor of Medicinal Chemistry, College of Pharmacy*

Bert N. La Du, Jr., M.D. — University of Michigan, Ph.D. — University of California, Berkeley, *Active Emeritus Professor of Pharmacology*

Fedor Medzihradsky, Ph.D. — Technische Hochschule, Munich, *Emeritus Professor of Biological Chemistry and Professor of Pharmacology*

Henry H. Swain, M.D. — University of Illinois, *Emeritus Professor of Pharmacology*

Wendell W. Weber, Ph.D. — Northwestern University, M.D. — University of Chicago, *Emeritus Professor of Pharmacology and Emeritus Professor of Toxicology, Environmental and Industrial Health, School of Public Health*

Vincent Zannoni, Ph.D. — George Washington University, *Emeritus Professor of Pharmacology and Emeritus Professor of Environmental and Industrial Health, School of Public Health*

Adjunct Faculty

Harvey R. Kaplan, Ph.D. — University of Connecticut, *Adjunct Professor of Pharmacology, Vice President of Scientific Affairs, Parke-Davis Pharmaceutical Research Division, Warner Lambert Company*

Roger S. Newton, Ph.D. — University of California, Davis, *Adjunct Associate Professor of Pharmacology and President and CEO Esperon Therapeutics*

Ronald Shebuski, Ph.D. — University of Minnesota, *Adjunct Professor of Pharmacology and Director, Cardiovascular Pharmacology, The Upjohn Company*

Kevin K.W. Wang, Ph.D. — University of British Columbia, *Adjunct Assistant Professor of Pharmacology and Senior Research Associate, Parke-Davis/Warner Lambert Pharmaceutical Research Division*

V. Research Faculty

Senior Research Scientist
Gail Winger, Ph.D., University of Michigan

Senior Associate Research Scientist
Gerald N. Levy, Ph.D., State University of New York
John R. Traynor, Ph.D., University of Aston

Assistant Research Scientists
Mary A. Bittner, Ph.D., University of Michigan
Marc A. Longino, Ph.D., University of Michigan
J. Kelly Bentley, Ph.D., Vanderbilt University
Ann E. Remmers, Ph.D., University of Michigan

Research Investigator
Ute M. Kent, Ph.D., Georgetown University

Lecturer
Martin M. Winbury, Ph.D., New York University

THE UNIVERSITY OF MICHIGAN

ARTES · SCIENTIA · VERITAS

MICHIGAN
MEDICAL SCHOOL

22

Future Prospects for Collaboration and the Dr. Maurice H. Seevers International Fellowship Fund

Paul F. Hollenberg, Ph.D.

It is certainly a pleasure to have this opportunity to make some comments regarding the Seevers Michigan Fellows in Pharmacology Program. I believe it is a truly outstanding, highly successful, and unique program which has been a superb model for international cooperation between scientists and has set the standard for this type of activity. Although I have had relatively limited involvement with this program so far, I look forward to future opportunities to get to know the many Japanese pharmacologists who are part of the Michigan family of scientists and to play a role in continuing the traditions developed over the years in this program; especially so because I have the honor of being the current Maurice H. Seevers Professor and Chair of Pharmacology here at the University of Michigan.

As I had a chance to review the thoughts and experiences of the members of the Michigan family who have contributed to this book, I was pleased to see the high level of enthusiasm expressed by all who have been involved in this remarkable enterprise. Although the Japanese scholars emphasized in their contributions the impact of the members of the University of Michigan Department of Pharmacology on the Japanese Fellows, it must be recognized that these outstanding scholars from Japan had profound impacts on the students, postdoctoral fellows and faculty of the Department of Pharmacology at the University of Michigan. Truly, in order for it to be as successful as it has been, there needed to be an exceptionally strong synergy and this obviously was the case. This program has not been a one way relationship in which only the visitors from Japan benefited. Clearly, the members of our department based in Ann Arbor learned much from their interactions with our Japanese colleagues and the ongoing research in the department benefited greatly from their remarkable abilities and tremendous hard work. The results emphatically demonstrate that the screening efforts performed prior to the acceptance of the fellows into this program were extremely effective and only the truly outstanding were selected to participate in this program. In addition to contributing directly to the success of the research projects performed in the department, the outstanding research performed by the fellows while in Ann Arbor greatly contributed to the national and international image of the department as an outstanding place to perform research. In addition to the significant contributions of the Michigan Fellows to our knowledge of pharmacology in the United States, they then went home and made remarkable contributions to the discipline of pharmacology in Japan, not only by their own research efforts, but by providing outstanding leadership for the development of the discipline in Japan.

Although this program was initially founded at a time when understanding between citizens of Japan and the United States was at a low level, this program contributed greatly to international understanding and fellowship and has served as an outstanding model for international cooperation between scientists. It is obvious from reading the accounts of members of the Michigan family from Japan as well as those based in Ann Arbor that this program began with cooperation in the laboratory which led to increased understanding and personal respect which was oftentimes followed by very intense friendships which profoundly affected the lives of the individuals involved. This was truly a triumph of the human spirit over misunderstanding, prejudice, and fear of the unknown. It is clear that as a direct result of this program many of the members of the Michigan Fellows have developed very special and intimate relationships with their counterparts at the University of Michigan and vice-versa.

The Michigan scholars now number more than 42 investigators. They have demonstrated a remarkable record of accomplishment as scientists and administrators and have played a major role in the development of pharmacology in Japan while at the same time contributing remarkably to the development of pharmacology in the Department of Pharmacology at the University of Michigan. Thus, the impact of the Seevers Michigan Fellows on pharmacology in both Japan and the United States has been profound. If Drs. Maurice Seevers and Walter Compton were able to see the success of this program which they so strongly believed in, they would not only be justifiably proud but, also in awe at what has been accomplished. One looks back in wonder at the incredible foresight and vision of these two individuals. At the same time we must also recognize Mr. Tsusai Sugawara for his outstanding support of this program.

By all measures the Michigan Fellows Program has been a tremendous success for all involved. As I look to the future, I hope to be able to play a more important role in fostering continuing interactions between Japanese scientists, the members of the Seevers Michigan Fellows and the members of the Department of Pharmacology based at the University of Michigan, to be able to expand the membership of this group, and to provide outstanding opportunities for the Japanese investigators who would like the opportunity to study in Ann Arbor. I hope that Ann Arbor will continue to be looked on as "a mecca for Japanese pharmacologists".

Finally, I would like to acknowledge Dr. Tomoji Yanagita for his strong support of this program as well as his efforts in the publication of this book. I should also like to acknowledge Dr. Edward F. Domino for his contributions over the years to this program as well as the critical role which he played in editing and publishing this book.

Appendices

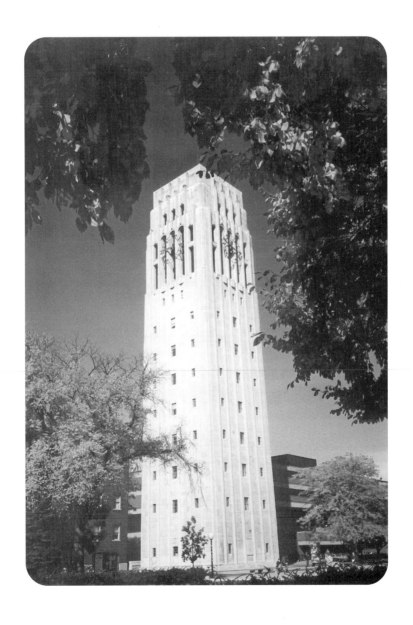

Appendix A: Seevers Fellows Biographical Sketches

Biographical Sketch

Fellow	Tai Akera, M.D., Ph.D.
Years in Michigan	U of M: 1962–1964 MSU: 1967–1970 1971–1987
Laboratory Mentor	Theodore M. Brody, Ph.D.
Primary Research Themes at UM	Biochemical pharmacology of opiate narcotics; phenothiazines and Na$^+$, K$^+$-ATPase

Post-Michigan Career		
	1964–1966	Instructor, Dept. of Pharmacology, Keio University School of Medicine
	1966–1971	Assistant Professor, Dept. of Pharmacology, Keio University School of Medicine
	1967–1970	Visiting Assistant Professor, Dept. of Pharmacology, Michigan State University
	1971–1974	Associate Professor, Dept. of Pharmacology, Michigan State University
	1974–1987	Professor, Dept. of Pharmacology, MSU
	1977–1978	Visiting Professor of Pharmacology, Tokai University School of Medicine
	1986–1987	Acting Chairman, Dept. of Pharmacology, Michigan State University
	1987–1991	Director, National Children's Hospital Medical Research Center
	1987–1997	Adjunct Professor, Tokai University School of Medicine
	1990–present	Adjunct Professor, Keio University School of Medicine
	1990–1991	Vice President, National Children's Hospital
	1991–1995	Vice President, and Director of Medical Research Center, Merck Research Laboratories

	1995–present	Head of Research and Development, Banyu Pharmaceutical Company
Public Service	1980–1984	Member, Biomedical Research Review Committee, National Institute of Drug Abuse
	1982–1984	Chairman, Gordon Research Conference on Cardiac Inotropic Agents
	1985–1989	Member, Pharmacology Study Section, National Institute of Health
	1987–present	Advisory Editor, Keio Journal of Medicine
	1990–1992	Editor-in-Chief, The Lancet Japanese Edition
	1991–present	Editor, Journal of Pharmacological and Toxicological Methods
	1995–present	Associate Editor, Pharmacological Reviews

Areas of Specialization   Cardiovascular pharmacology; physiology and biochemistry of heart muscle; drug development

Biographical Sketch

Fellow	Toru Endo, Ph.D.
Years in Michigan	1994–1995
Laboratory Mentor	Charles B. Smith, M.D., Ph.D.
Primary Research Theme at UM	Effects of α_2 agonists on 5–HT release from hippocampus and dorsal raphé slices in morphine dependent rats

Post-Michigan Career	1996–present	Assistant Professor, Department of Pharmacology, Faculty of Pharmaceutical Sciences, Health Sciences University of Hokkaido
Public Service	1996–present	Member of The Japanese Pharmacological Society
	1997–present	Member of the Japanese Society of Toxicological Sciences
	1997–present	Member of The Japanese Neurochemical Society
	1998–present	Certified pharmacist of The Japanese Society of Clinical Pharmacology and Therapeutics

Areas of Specialization	Neuropharmacology; gastrointestinal pharmacology

Biographical Sketch

Fellow	Naohisa Fukuda, Ph.D.
Years at Michigan	1981–1982
Laboratory Mentor	Edward F. Domino, M.D.
Primary Research Theme at UM	EEG effects of phencyclidine and ketamine

Post-Michigan Career	1982–1985	Research Scientist, Dept. of CNS Pharmacology, Biology Research Laboratories, Central Research Division, Takeda Chemical Industries, Ltd.
	1985–1993	Senior Research Scientist, Dept. of CNS Pharmacology, Pharmaceutical Research Laboratories I, Research and Development Division, Takeda Chemical Industries, Ltd.

1993–present   Manager, Quality Assurance, Good Clinical
                                          Practice, Regulatory Affairs Department,
                                          Pharmaceutical Group, Takeda Chemical
                                          Industries, Ltd.

Areas of Specialization   Antianxiety drugs; brain ischemia; neurodegenerative diseases

Biographical Sketch

Fellow	Takeo Fukuda, M.D., Ph.D.
Years at Michigan	1968–1969
Laboratory Mentor	Julian Villarreal, M.D., Ph.D
Primary Research Theme at UM	Behavioral pharmacology

Post-Michigan Career	1966–1968	Research Associate, Dept. of Pharmacology, Kyushu University Faculty of Medicine
	1968–1971	Instructor, Dept. of Pharmacology, Kyushu University Faculty of Medicine
	1971–1977	Associate Professor, Dept. of Pharmacology, Kyushu University Faculty of Medicine
	1977–present	Professor, Dept. of Pharmacology, Kagoshima University Faculty of Medicine
	1981–1983	Director, Institute of Laboratory Animal Science, Kagoshima University Faculty of Medicine
	1991–1993	Dean of Faculty of Medicine, Kagoshima University
Public Service	1976–1982	Member, Financial Committee, Japanese Pharmacological Society
	1978–1979	Member, Student Welfare Committee, Kagoshima University
	1979–1980	Member, Student Guidance Committee, Kagoshima University
	1989–1993	Board of Trustees, Kagoshima University
	1990–1994	Member, Financial Committee, Japanese Pharmacological Society
	1992–present	Member, Japanese Society for Pharmacoanesthesiology
	1993–present	Board of Directors, Japanese Society of Neuropsychopharmacology
	1994–present	Board of Directors, Japanese Pharmacological Society
	1996–1997	President, Japanese Society of Neuropsychopharmacology
Area of Specialization	Neuropharmacology	

Biographical Sketch

Fellow	Tatsuo Furukawa, M.D., Ph.D.	
Years at Michigan	1961–1963	
Laboratory Mentor	Theodore M. Brody, Ph.D.	
Primary Research Theme at UM	Mechanisms involved in CCl_4 toxicity	
Post-Michigan Career	1963–1964	Instructor, Dept. of Pharmacology, Kyushu University Faculty of Medicine
	1964–1967	Associate Professor, Dept. of Pharmacology, Wakayama Medical College
	1967–1968	Associate Professor, Dept. of Pharmacology, Kurume University School of Medicine
	1968–1974	Professor, Dept. of Pharmacology, Fukuoka University School of Pharmaceutical Sciences
	1974–1997	Professor, Dept. of Pharmacology, Fukuoka University School of Medicine
	1988–1993	Dean, Postgraduate courses, Fukuoka University School of Medicine
	1993–1994	Dean, Nursing School, Fukuoka University
	1997–present	Emeritus Professor, Dept. of Pharmacology, Fukuoka University School of Medicine
Public Service	1982–1986	Editor, Japanese Journal of Pharmacology
	1987–1988	President, Japanese Pharmacological Society
	1994–1995	President, Japanese Society of Neuropsychopharmacology
Scientific Meetings Hosted	1981	Ninth Symposium on Psychoneuropharmacology
	1981	Fourth Symposium on Sulphur Amino Acids
	1983	Twelfth Symposium on Drug Activity
	1988	Sixty-First Meeting of the Japanese Pharmacological Society
	1991	Tenth Japan-Korea Joint Seminar on Pharmacology
	1995	Twenty-Fifth Annual Meeting of the Japanese Society of Neuropsychopharmacology
Honors and Prizes	1972	Kanae Award for Medical Research
Areas of Specialization	Neuropsychopharmacology; nonadrenergic, noncholinergic, and cholinergic control of autonomic nerves; renin-angiotensin system in the brain	

Biographical Sketch

Fellow	Eiichi Hasegawa, M.D., Ph.D.
Years at Michigan	1969–1970
Laboratory Mentors	Charles B. Smith, M.D., Ph.D. T. R. Tephly, Ph.D.
Primary Research Theme at UM	Autonomic pharmacology and drug metabolism

Post-Michigan Career	1971–1978	Professor, Dept. of Pharmacology, Kyoto Prefectural Medical College
	1978–1989	Board of Directors, The Green Cross Corporation, Ltd.
	Present	Dean, Sakura City College of International Studies
Public Service	Present	Japan P.E.N. Club
	Present	Sakura Rotary Club

Area of Specialization	Neuropharmacology

Biographical Sketch

Fellow	Shiro Hisada, M.D., Ph.D.
Years at Michigan	1961–1962
Laboratory Mentor	Donald R. Bennett, M.D., Ph.D.
Primary Research Theme at UM	Cardiovascular pharmacology

Post-Michigan Career	1952–1979	Professor, Dept. of Pharmacology, Nagoya City Municipal University School of Medicine
	1969–1971	Dean, School of Medicine, Nagoya Municipal University
	1979–present	Professor Emeritus, Nagoya City University
Public Service	1965–1966	President, Japanese Pharmacological Society
	1969–1979	Medical Inspector, Japan Ministry of Education
Honors	1981–present	Honorary Member, Japanese Pharmacological Society

Areas of Specialization	Brain amino acids; release of antidiuretic hormone

Biographical Sketch

Fellow	*Eikichi Hosoya, M.D., Ph.D.
Years at Michigan	1952–1954
Laboratory Mentors	Theodore M. Brody, Ph.D. Lauren A. Woods, M.D., Ph.D.
Primary Research Theme at UM	Papillary muscle phosphorous/oxygen ratios; morphine biotransformation

Post-Michigan Career

1955	Associate Professor of Pharmacology, Keio University Medical School
1963–1974	Professor and Chairman, Department of Pharmacology, Keio University Medical School
1974–1996	Emeritus Professor of Pharmacology, Keio University Medical School
1974–1978	Kanebo Pharmaceutical Co.
1978–1996	Director of Research and Development, Tsumura Pharmaceutical Co.

Public Service

1963–1973	Editorial Board, Japanese Journal of Pharmacology
1963–1973	Editorial Board, Folia Pharmacologica Japonica
1970–1980	Advisory Board, Pharmacological Communications
1979–1992	Editorial Board, Trends in Pharmacological Sciences
1965–1977	Member, WHO Expert Panel on Drug Abuse
1970–1971	President, Japanese Pharmacological Society
1971–1980	Member, International Advisory Board of IUPHAR
1975–1976	Second Vice President, IUPHAR

Areas of Specialization	Opioid pharmacology; drugs of abuse; active substances in traditional Chinese medicines

*Deceased

Biographical Sketch

Fellow	Shoichi Iida, M.D., Ph.D.
Years at Michigan	1961–1963
Laboratory Mentor	Gerald A. Deneau, Ph.D.
Primary Research Theme at UM	Tolerance to and dependence on alcohol in monkeys

Post-Michigan Career	1963–1968	Associate Professor, Dept. of Pharmacology, Hokkaido University School of Medicine
	1968–1987	Professor, Dept. of Pharmacology, Hokkaido University School of Dentistry
	1987–present	Professor Emeritus, Hokkaido University
	Present	Manager, Research Forum of Officers on Collaborative Program in Industry and Universities in Hokkaido
Honors	1988–present	Honorary Member, Basic Dental Medical Society
	1992–present	Honorary Member, Japanese Pharmacological Society

Areas of Specialization	Drug dependence; cardiac glycoside receptors

Biographical Sketch

Fellow	Fumio Ikomi, M.D., Ph.D.
Years at Michigan	1968–1970
Laboratory Mentor	James H. Woods, Ph.D.
Primary Research Theme at UM	Reinforcing property of ethanol

Post-Michigan Career	1970–1979	Lecturer, Shinshu University School of Medicine
	1979–1984	Director, Suwa Kohan Hospital
	1985–1992	Director, Kofu City Hospital

Public Service	1985–1992	Board of Directors, Kofu Doctors' Society
	1985–1992	Board of Directors, Yamanashi Public Health Hospital
	1985–1992	Board of Directors, Yamanashi Medical Society
Scientific Meetings Hosted	1990	Congress of Clinical Studies on Anti-Cancer Drugs
Honors	1992	Kofu Mayor's Outstanding Effort Award
Areas of Specialization		Alcohol dependence; clinical pharmacology of respiratory organ system; therapeutics in elderly patients

Biographical Sketch

Fellow	Reizo Inoki, M.D., Ph.D.
Years at Michigan	1963–1965
Laboratory Mentor	Gerald A. Deneau, Ph.D.
Primary Research Theme at UM	Self-administration of nicotine

Post-Michigan Career	1967–1988	Lecturer, Nara Medical College
	1969–1988	Lecturer, School of Medicine, Osaka University
	1975–1978	Lecturer, Fukuoka Dental College
	1978–1993	Professor, Dept. of Pharmacology, Osaka University Faculty of Dentistry
	1984–1988	Lecturer, School of Dentistry, Nagasaki University
	1988–present	Guest Professor, Xian Military Medical
	1989–1993	Dean, Faculty of Dentistry, Osaka University College
	1994–present	Professor Emeritus, Osaka University
	1994–1995	Lecturer, Shiga Medical College
	1994–present	Head, Okanami General Hospital
Public Service	1981–1983	Board Member, Osaka University
	1986–1988	Member, Executive Committee, International Narcotic Research Conference
	1991–1992	President, Japanese Society for the Study of Pain
	1992–1994	Board of Trustees, Japanese Pharmacological Society
	1993–1994	Member, Educational Committee in the Ministry of Education
Scientific Meetings Hosted	1984	Fifth Analgesics-Opioid Peptides Symposium
	1985	Ninth Symposium of the Pharmacological Sciences of the Japan Science Council
	1985	Sixty-eighth Kinki Area Pharmacological Meeting of the Japanese Pharmacological Society
	1991	International Symposium Processing and Inhibition of Nociceptive Information
	1992	Sixteenth Annual Meeting of Japan Neuroscience Society
Areas of Specialization		Action of opioid peptides; mechanism of action of analgesics

Biographical Sketch

Fellow	*Hiroshi Ito, M.D., Ph.D.
Years at Michigan	1965–1966
Laboratory Mentor	Lloyd Beck, Ph.D.
Primary Research Theme at UM	Autonomic pharmacology
Post-Michigan Career	1967–1976 Professor, Dept. of Pharmacology, Yokohama City University School of Medicine
Areas of Specialization	Cardiovascular pharmacology; kidney cell membrane functions

Biographical Sketch

Fellow	*Teiji Iwami, M.D., Ph.D.
Years at Michigan	1966–1968
Laboratory Mentor	Henry H. Swain, M.D.
Primary Research Theme at UM	Cardiovascular pharmacology
Post-Michigan Career	1968–1973 Associate Professor, Dept. of Pharmacology, Hirosaki University School of Medicine 1973–1983 Professor, Dept. of Pharmacology, Hirosaki University School of Medicine
Areas of Specialization	Pharmacology of coronary artery drugs; fluorine poisoning; experimental hypertension

*Deceased

Biographical Sketch

Fellow	Shin-ichi Iwata, M.D., Ph.D.	
Years at Michigan	1993–1995	
Laboratory Mentor	Margaret Gnegy, Ph.D.	
Primary Research Theme at UM	Amphetamine sensitization	
Post-Michigan Career	1995–present	Assistant Professor, Dept. of Pharmacology, Faculty of Medicine, Kagoshima University
Public Service	1984–present	Member, Japanese Society of Neurology
	1987–present	Member, Japanese Pharmacological Society
	1987–present	Member, Japanese Society of Neuropsychopharmacology
Area of Specialization	Neuropsychopharmacology	

Biographical Sketch

Fellow	Hiroshi Kaneto, Ph.D.
Years at Michigan	1959–1960
Laboratory Mentor	Lauren A. Woods, M.D., Ph.D.
Primary Research Theme at UM	Morphine receptor binding

Post-Michigan Career

1960–1967	Research Assistant, Dept. of Pharmacology, Osaka University Faculty of Pharmaceutical Sciences
1967–1969	Associate Professor, Osaka Pharmaceutical College
1969–1996	Professor, Dept. of Pharmacology, Nagasaki University Faculty of Pharmaceutical Sciences
1990–1992	Dean, Faculty of Pharmaceutical Sciences, Nagasaki University
1996–present	Emeritus Professor of Pharmacology, Nagasaki University

Public Service

1965–present	Member, Board of Trustees, and Director, Japanese Pharmacological Society
1976–1995	Board of Trustees, Pharmaceutical Society of Japan
1981–1996	Board of Trustees then Directors, Japanese Society of Neuropsychopharmacology (JSNP)
1984–1990	Editor of Society's journal, JSNP
1985–1993	Editor-in-Chief, J. Pharmacobio-Dyn. PSJ
1990–1996	Board of Trustees then Directors, Japanese Society for the Study of Pain
1990–present	Board of Trustees, Journal Editor, Japanese Medical Society on Alcohol Studies
1993–1995	Board of Consulting Editors, Bulletin Publication, PSJ
1995–1996	President, Japanese Pharmacological Society
1996–1997	President, Japanese Society for the Study of Pain

Scientific Meetings Hosted

1971–1995	Five symposia and two regional scientific meetings of the Japanese Pharmacological Society and the Pharmaceutical Society of Japan
1996	Sixty-ninth Annual Scientific Meeting of the Japanese Pharmacological Society

Areas of Specialization	Drug tolerance and dependence; narcotic analgesics and pain mechanisms

Biographical Sketch

Fellow	*Nobuo Katsuda, M.D., Ph.D.
Years at Michigan	1963–1965
Laboratory Mentor	Edward F. Domino, M.D.
Primary Research Theme at UM	Electrophysiology
Post-Michigan Career	Since returning to Japan in 1965 Dr. N. Katsuda was:
	Associate Professor, Dept. of Pharmacology, Kyushu University Faculty of Medicine
	Professor, Dept. of Pharmacology, Kyushu University Faculty of Dentistry
	Professor Emeritus, Kyushu University
Honors	Honorary Member, Basic Dental Medical Society
	Honorary Member, Japanese Pharmacological Society
Areas of Specialization	CNS pharmacology; electrophysiology

Biographical Sketch

Fellow	Shiroh Kishioka, M.D., Ph.D.	
Years at Michigan	1995–1997	
Laboratory Mentor	James H. Woods, Ph.D.	
Primary Research Theme at UM	Respiratory effects of opioids	
Post-Michigan Career	1997–present	Professor, Dept. of Pharmacology, Wakayama Medical College
Public Service	1997–present	Committee Member, Japanese Narcotics Research Conference
Area of Specialization	Neuropharmacology; behavioral pharmacology	

*Deceased

Biographical Sketch

Fellow	Izuru Matsuoka, M.D., Ph.D.
Years at Michigan	1968–1970
Laboratory Mentor	Edward F. Domino, M.D.
Primary Research Theme at UM	Cholinergic and vestibular pharmacology

Post-Michigan Career	1970–1978	Assistant, Department of Otolaryngology, Kyoto University Faculty of Medicine
	1978–1985	Instructor, Department of Otolaryngology, Kyoto University Faculty of Medicine
	1985–1993	Chief, Otolaryngology, Shizuoka General Hospital
	1993–1995	Director, Nagisa Hospital

Area of Specialization	Vestibular pharmacology

Biographical Sketch

Fellow	Kichihiko Matsusaki, M.D., Ph.D.
Years at Michigan	1967–1968
Laboratory Mentor	Henry H. Swain, M.D.
Primary Research Theme at UM	Electrophysiology of cardiac muscle cells

Post-Michigan Career	1968–1970	Associate Professor, Dept. of Pharmacology, Kagoshima University Faculty of Medicine
	1970–1980	Professor, Ryukyu University School of Medicine
	1980–1986	Vice–president, Miyazaki Medical School
	1986–1990	Professor, Kagoshima Women's Colle⌐

Area of Specialization	Developmental pharmacology

Biographical Sketch

Fellow	Masaru Minami, M.D., Ph.D.
Years at Michigan	1985–1986
Laboratory Mentor	Benedict R. Lucchesi, M.D., Ph.D.
Primary Research Theme at UM	Cardiovascular pharmacology

Post-Michigan Career

1985–1986	Associate Professor, Dept. of Pharmacology, Hokkaido University (Higashi Nippon-Gakuen University) School of Medicine
1986–present	Chairman and Professor, Dept. of Pharmacology, Health Sciences University of Hokkaido Faculty of Pharmaceutical Sciences

Public Service

1986, at various times to present	Councilor and member of Japanese Pharmacological Association Japanese Society of Clinical Pharmacology and Therapeutics Society for Spontaneously Hypertensive Rats Chairman, Hokkaido Branch, Pharmaceutical Society of Japan Editorial Board, Biogenic Amines and Journal of Toxicological Sciences

Area of Specialization   Integration of autonomic nervous system, especially studies related to catecholamines and serotonin

Biographical Sketch

Fellow	*Matué Miyasaka, M.D., Ph.D.	
Years at Michigan	1966–1968	
Laboratory Mentor	Edward F. Domino, M.D.	
Primary Research Theme at UM	Electrophysiological research on the brain and drug action	
Post-Michigan Career	1968–1974	Lecturer, Dept. of Psychiatry, Tokyo Medical and Dental University School of Medicine
	1974–1996	Chairman, Professor, Dept. of Psychiatry, Dokkyo University School of Medicine
Public Service	1984 to present at various times	President then member Board of Directors, Japanese Society of Epilepsy
		President then member Board of Directors, Japanese Society of Geriatric Psychiatry
		President then member Board of Directors, Japanese Society of Psychiatry and Neurology
		Board of Directors, Japanese Society of EEG and EMG
		Japan Epilepsy Research Foundation
		Board of Directors, Japanese Society of Biological Psychiatry
	1995	Vice–president, International Meeting of EMG and Clinical Neurophysiology
Honors	1970	Schimazaki's Prize for Psychiatric Research
Areas of Specialization	Clinical estimation (rating) of the effects of nootropic drugs, antiepileptics, and psychotropic drugs; neuropharmacology and quantitative EEG research	

*Deceased

Biographical Sketch

Fellow	Sadao Miyata, M.D.
Years at Michigan	1964–1965
Laboratory Mentor	Theodore M. Brody, Ph.D.
Primary Research Theme at UM	Determination of catecholamines in blood

Post-Michigan Career	1967–1977	Professor, Dept. of Pharmacology, Kyoto College of Pharmacy
	1977–1991	Professor, Dept. of Pharmacology, Hyogo College of Medicine
	1991–present	Professor Emeritus, Hyogo College of Medicine
Scientific Meetings Hosted	1970	President, Kinki Meeting of Japanese Pharmacological Society

Areas of Specialization Autocoids (kinin-like substances); vascular smooth muscle; drug metabolism

Biographical Sketch

Fellow	Tadashi Murano, M.D., Ph.D.
Years at Michigan	1962–1963
Laboratory Mentor	Theodore M. Brody, Ph.D.
Primary Research Theme at UM	Na$^+$, K$^+$, Mg^{++} activated ATPase

Post-Michigan Career	1963–1970	Professor, Dept. of Pharmacology, Wakayama Medical College
	1970–1978	President, Wakayama Medical College
	1978–1987	Executive Managing Director, Pharmaceutical Division, Hoechst Japan Company, Ltd.
	1987–1993	Medical Advisor in charge of Ciba Vision Division, Ciba-Geigy Ltd.
Honors	1987–present	Honorary Member, Japanese Pharmacological Society
	1992–present	Honorary Member, Japanese Society of Toxicological Sciences

Area of Specialization Biochemical pharmacology

Biographical Sketch

Fellow	Kengo Nakai, M.D., Ph.D.
Years at Michigan	1959–1960
Laboratory Mentor	Gerald A. Deneau, Ph.D.
Primary Research Theme at UM	Meperidine metabolism

Post-Michigan Career		
	1960–1971	Associate Professor, Sapporo Medical College
	1971–1990	Professor, Dept. of Pharmacology, Akita University School of Medicine
	1972–1976	Director, Medical Library, Akita University
	1976–1980	Dean, Akita University School of Medicine
	1981–1982	Dean of Students, Akita University
	1990–present	Professor Emeritus, Akita University

Areas of Specialization	Drug metabolism; toxicology

Biographical Sketch

Fellow	Yoshihisa Nakai, M.D., Ph.D.
Years at Michigan	1966–1968
Laboratory Mentor	Edward F. Domino, M.D.
Primary Research Theme at UM	Effect of psychoactive drugs on auditory and visual pathways

Post-Michigan Career		
	1968–1973	Assistant, Dept. of Pharmacology, Kyoto University School of Medicine
	1973–1975	Instructor, Dept. of Otolaryngology, Kyoto University-Hospital
	1975–present	Director, Nakai ENT Clinic

Public Service		
	1960–present	Member, Japanese Otorhinolaryngological Society
	1962–1993	Member, Japanese Pharmacological Society

Area of Specialization	Electrophysiological study of central nervous system depressants

Biographical Sketch

Fellow	Tetsuo Oka, Ph.D.
Years at Michigan	1967–1969
Laboratory Mentor	Carl C. Hug, Jr., M.D., Ph.D.
Primary Research Theme at UM	Opiate receptor binding and uptake

Post-Michigan Career

1964–1971	Instructor, Dept. of Pharmacology, School of Medicine, Keio University
1972–1974	Assistant Professor, Dept. of Pharmacology, School of Medicine, Keio University
1974	Associate Professor, Dept. of Pharmacology, School of Medicine, Keio University
1974–present	Professor and Chairman, Dept. of Pharmacology, School of Medicine, Tokai University

Area of Specialization   Endogenous opioid peptides

Biographical Sketch

Fellow	Toru Otani, M.D.
Years at Michigan	1969–1971
Laboratory Mentor	Henry H. Swain, M.D.
Primary Research Theme at UM	Cardiovascular pharmacology
Post-Michigan Career	Founder and Director of the Otani Medical Clinic and Hospital, as well as Chitose Airport Clinic

Biographical Sketch

Fellow	Katsuharu Saito, M.D., Ph.D.
Years at Michigan	1996–1997
Laboratory Mentor	Benedict R. Lucchesi, M.D., Ph.D.
Primary Research Theme at UM	Antiarrhythmic effects of new class III antiarrhythmics

Post-Michigan Career

1997–1998	Department of Cardiovascular Medicine, Hokkaido University School of Medicine
1998–present	Cardiologist, Touei Hospital

Area of Specialization   Cardiovascular pharmacology; cardiovascular medicine

Biographical Sketch

Fellow	Akira Sakuma, Ph.D.
Years at Michigan	1958–1960
Laboratory Mentor	Lloyd Beck, Ph.D.
Primary Research Theme at UM	Reflex dilatation in dog hindquarters

Post-Michigan Career	1959–1960	Assistant Professor, Dept. of Pharmacology, University of Tokyo Faculty of Medicine
	1960–1995	Visiting Lecturer, Dept. of Pharmacology, Tokyo Women's College of Medicine
	1963–1973	Associate Professor, Dept. of Pharmacology, Institute for Cardiovascular Diseases, Tokyo Medical and Dental University
	1969–1970	Geigy S.A. Visiting Professor, Dept. of Internal Medicine, University of Basle/Scientific Calculating Center
	1974–1996	Professor, Dept. of Clinical Pharmacology, Division of Information Medicine, Medical Research Institute, Tokyo Medical and Dental University
Public Service	1997–present	Senior Counselor, Organization for Pharmaceutical Safety and Research
	1968–1994	Central Advisory Board Member for the Japanese Ministry of Health and Education
	1980–present	Board Member, Japanese Society of Clinical Pharmacology and Therapeutics
	1981–1995	Board Member, Japan Region of the Biometric Society
	1988–1992	Council Member, International Society of Clinical Pharmacology and Therapeutics
	1989–1990	President, Japanese Society of Clinical Pharmacology and Therapeutics
	1990–1993	President, Japan Region of the Biometric Society
	1992–1995	Council Member, International Biometric Society
Area of Specialization	Design and analysis of clinical trials	

Biographical Sketch

Fellow	*Kiro Shimamoto, M.D., Ph.D.
Years at Michigan	1960–1961
Laboratory Mentor	Henry H. Swain, M.D.
Primary Research Theme at UM	Cardiovascular pharmacology

Post-Michigan Career	1958–1968	Professor, Dept. of Pharmacology, Kyoto University Faculty of Medicine
	1968–1972	Director, Biology Research Laboratories, Takeda Chemical Industry, Ltd.
	1972–1982	Board of Directors, Takeda Chemical Industry, Limited
	1974–1994	Professor Emeritus, Kyoto University
Public Service	1962–1968	Board of Directors, Japanese Pharmacological Society
Honors	1974–1994	Honorary Member, Japanese Pharmacological Society

Areas of Specialization	Autonomic pharmacology; toxicological sciences

Biographical Sketch

Fellow	Yuji Sudo, D.V.M., Ph.D.	
Years at Michigan	1994–1995	
Laboratory Mentor	Benedict R. Lucchesi, M.D., Ph.D.	
Primary Research Theme at UM	Thrombosis	
Post-Michigan Career	1995–present	Senior Research Manager, Biology Research Lab., Fujisawa Pharmaceutical Co., Ltd.
Area of Specialization	Cardiovascular pharmacology; organ transplantation	

*Deceased

Biographical Sketch

Fellow	Sakutaro Tadokoro, M.D., Ph.D.
Years of Stay	1965–1967
Laboratory Mentor	Julian Villareal, M.D., Ph.D.
Primary Research Theme	Behavioral pharmacology using monkeys

Post-Michigan Career	1959–1972	Associate Professor, Dept. of Pharmacology, Gunma University School of Medicine
	1972–1992	Professor, Dept. of Pharmacology, Gunma University School of Medicine
	1983–1985	Director, Institute of Experimental Animals, Gunma University School of Medicine
	1985–1989	Dean of Student Affairs, Gunma University
	1985–1989	Director of Health Center, Gunma University
	1985–1989	Councilor, Gunma University
	1992–present	Professor Emeritus, Gunma University
	1993–present	President, Gunma Prefectural College of Health Sciences
Public Service	1974–1989	Editor, Pharmacology Biochemical Behavior
	1978–1979	President, Japanese Medical Society of Alcohol Studies
	1981–present	Member, Central Drug Affairs Committee, Ministry of Health and Welfare
	1982–present	Chairman, Environmental Council Committee, Maebashi City
	1982–1986	President, Alumni Association, Gunma University School of Medicine
	1983–1986	Chairman, Board of Directors, Japanese Association of Neuropsychopharmacology
	1989–1990	President, Japanese Society of Neuropsychopharmacology
Honors	1992–present	Honorary Member, Japanese Medical Society of Alcohol Studies
	1992–present	Honorary Member, Japanese Society of Neuropsychopharmacology
Areas of Specialization		Behavioral pharmacology; drug dependence; nursing and medical care

Biographical Sketch

Fellow	Kohji Takada, Ph.D.
Years at Michigan	1983–1985
Laboratory Mentor	James H. Woods, Ph.D.
Primary Research Theme at UM	Mechanisms mediating anxiogenic and aversive drug effects

Post-Michigan Career	1985–1986	Visiting Fellow, NIDA Addiction Research Center
	1987–1996	Senior Research Scientist, Preclinical Research Division, Central Institute for Experimental Animals
	1991–present	Lecturer, Dept. Of Psychology, Keio University
	1996–1997	Member, Research Center Research and Development, Gleran Pharmaceutical Co., Ltd.
	1997–present	Associate Scientist, Worldwide Scientific Affairs, Philip Morris K.K.
Public Service	1975–present	Councilor, Japanese Pharmaceutical Society
	1981–present	Japanese Society of Neuropsychopharmacology and Member, Committee on General Affairs,
	1990–1996	Vice–President, International Study Group Investigating Drugs as Reinforcers
	1992–present	Member, Organizing Committee, Young Researcher's Society of Neurobehavioral Pharmacology
Honors	1984	Student Travel Award, ISGIDAR
	1993	International Visiting Scientists and Technical Exchange Program Travel Award, NIDA
Areas of Specialization	Behavioral pharmacology; drug dependence	

Biographical Sketch

Fellow	Shuji Takaori, M.D., Ph.D.
Years at Michigan	1959–1961
Laboratory Mentor	Gerald A. Deneau, Ph.D.
Primary Research Theme at UM	Effects of CNS drugs on EEG

Post-Michigan Career	1962–1972	Associate Professor, Dept. of Pharmacology, Kyoto University Faculty of Medicine
	1972–1990	Professor, Dept. of Pharmacology, Kyoto
	1990–1994	Vice–President for Academic Affairs, Shimane Medical University
	1991–present	Professor Emeritus of Kyoto University Faculty of Medicine
	1994–present	President, Shimane Medical University
Public Service	1970–present	Councilor, Japanese Society of Clinical Pharmacology and Therapeutics
	1973–present	Councilor, Japanese Society of Toxicological Science
	1974–1978, 1980–1984, 1986–1990	Board of Trustees, Japanese Pharmacological Society
	1979–present	Councilor, Japan Society for Equilibrium Research
	1981–1986, 1989–1993	Board of Trustees, Japanese Society of Neuropsychopharmacology
	1982–present	Councilor, Japanese Society of Electro-encephalography and Electromyography
	1983–1987	Board of Trustees, Japanese Medical Society of Alcohol Studies
	1989–1993	Board of Trustees, Japanese Medical Society of Alcohol Studies
	1985	President, Japanese Society of Neuropsycho-pharmacology
	1986–present	Councilor, Japanese Society for Ocular Pharmacology
	1988–1989	President, Japanese Pharmacological Society
	1988–present	Member, Collegium Internationale of Neuropsychopharmacologicum
Honors	1993	Honorary Member, Japanese Pharmacological Society
Areas of Specialization		Site of action of central drugs; studies on central monoamines; mechanism of epilepsy; studies on vestibular mechanism

Biographical Sketch

Fellow	*Tsuneyoshi Tanabe, M.D., Ph.D.
Years at Michigan	1956–1957
Laboratory Mentor	Edward J. Cafruny, M.D., Ph.D.
Primary Research Theme at UM	Adrenal hypertrophy in rats treated with morphine; diuretic action of drugs injected into the renal artery of dogs

Post-Michigan Career	1957–1975	Professor, Dept. of Pharmacology, Hokkaido University School of Medicine
	1969–1970	Dean, School of Medicine, Hokkaido University
	1975–1996	Professor Emeritus, Hokkaido University
	1975–1993	Professor, Dept. of Pharmacology, Higashi-Nippon-Gakuen University Faculty of Pharmaceutical Sciences
	1993–1996	Professor Emeritus, Higashi-Nippon-Gakuen University

Public Service	1985	Trustee, Higashi-Nippon-Gakuen University
	1969–1972	Expert Member, Scientific Council of the Minister of Education

Areas of Specialization	Experimental and clinical pharmacology

Biographical Sketch

Fellow	Hiroko Togashi, Ph.D.
Years at Michigan	1996
Laboratory Mentor	Charles B. Smith, M.D., Ph.D.
Primary Research Theme at UM	Neurotransmitter release mechanisms modulated by opioid receptors

Post-Michigan Career	1996–present	Assistant Professor, Dept. of Pharmacology, Graduate School of Medicine, Hokkaido University

Area of Specialization	Neuropharmacology

*Deceased

Biographical Sketch

Fellow	Akira Tsujimoto, M.D., Ph.D.
Years at Michigan	1965–1967
Laboratory Mentors	Roy Hudson, Ph.D. Charles C. Hug, Jr. M.D., Ph.D.
Primary Research Theme at UM	CNS pharmacology; pharmacology of nicotine

Post-Michigan Career

1965–1968	Associate Professor, Dept. of Pharmacology, Nara Medical University
1967–1969	Lecturer, Osaka University School of Dentistry
1968–1991	Professor, Dept. of Pharmacology, Hiroshima University School of Dentistry
1974–present	Lecturer, Nara Medical University
1982–1984	Director, Medical Science Branch Library, Hiroshima University
1985–1986	Lecturer, Kagoshima University School
1986–1988	Dean, Hiroshima University School of Medicine
1990–1991	Lecturer, Nagasaki University School of Dentistry
1991–present	Director, Yuno Hot-Spring Hospital
1991–1994	Lecturer, Hiroshima University School of Dentistry
1991–present	Professor Emeritus of Hiroshima University
1992–1993	Lecturer, Kagoshima University School of Dentistry
1992–present	Lecturer, Kinki University School of Medicine

Public Service

1980–1982, 1988–1990	Member, Hiroshima University Senate
1986–1988	Member, Medical Council of Hiroshima Prefecture
1988–1991	Board of Directors, Japanese Association for Oral Biology

Areas of Specialization   Nicotine; catecholamines, uptake, storage release; cyclic AMP; prostaglandins

Biographical Sketch

Fellow	*Showa Ueki, M.D., Ph.D.
Years at Michigan	1957–1959
Laboratory Mentor	Edward F. Domino, M.D.
Primary Research Theme at UM	Limbic system and spinal cord pharmacology

Post-Michigan Career	1959–1966	Associate Professor, Dept. of Pharmacology, Kyushu University Faculty of Medicine
	1966–1990	Professor, Dept. of Pharmacology, Kyushu University Faculty of Medicine
	1990–1993	Professor Emeritus, Kyushu University
	1990–1993	Adjunct Professor, Fukuoka University School of Medicine
Public Service	1980–1981	President, Japanese Pharmacological Society
	1985–1990	Member, Central Advisory Committee on New Drugs, Ministry of Health and Welfare
	1988–1989	President, Japanese Society of Neuropsychopharmacology
	1991–1993	Chairman, Board of Directors, Japanese Society of Neuropsychopharmacology
Honors and Prizes	1984	Academy Prize of Japanese Society of Pharmaceutical Sciences
Areas of Specialization	CNS and behavioral pharmacology; pharmacology of cannabis	

*Deceased

Biographical Sketch

Fellow	Ken-ichi Yamamoto, Ph.D.	
Years at Michigan	1963–1965	
Laboratory Mentor	Edward F. Domino, M.D.	
Primary Research Theme at UM	EEG, sleep, and cholinergic mechanisms	
Post-Michigan Career	1965–1996	Staff, Dept. of Pharmacology, Shionogi Research Laboratories (Member since 1952)
	1970–1972	Lecturer, Shinshu University School of Medicine
	1973–1988	Director, Division of Neuropharmacology, Shionogi Research Laboratories
	1988–1996	Managing Director, The Cell Science Research Foundation and Staff, Shionogi Research Laboratories
	1989–1997	Advisor, Hokurikuseiyake, Co., Ltd., Research Division
Public Service	1968–present	Member, Japanese Pharmacological Society
	1972–present	Member, Japanese EEG and EMG Society
	1974–present	Member, Pharmacometrics
	1980–present	Member, Japan Neuroscience Society
	1985–present	Member, Japan Neuropsychopharmacology Society
	1986–present	Member, Collegium Internationale Neuropsychopharmacologicum
Areas of Specialization	Drug dependence; preclinical studies on drugs; EEG analysis of brain mechanisms	

Biographical Sketch

Fellow	Tsuneyuki Yamamoto, Ph.D.
Years at Michigan	1982–1984; 1988
Laboratory Mentor	James H. Woods, Ph.D.
Primary Research Theme at UM	Drug discrimination

Post-Michigan Career	1975–1990	Assistant, Dept. of Pharmacology, Kyushu University Faculty of Pharmaceutical Sciences
	1990–present	Associate Professor, Dept. of Pharmacology, Kyushu University Faculty of Pharmaceutical Sciences
Public Service	1985–present	Member, Pharmaceutical Society of Japan Councilor, Japanese Pharmacological Society Councilor and Trustee, Japanese Society of Neuropsychopharmacology
Honors	1995	Scientific Award, Japanese Society of Neuropsychopharmacology
Areas of Specialization		Behavioral pharmacology; learning and memory; preclinical studies on psychotherapeutic drugs

Biographical Sketch

Fellow	Tomoji Yanagita, M.D., Ph.D.
Years at Michigan	1960–1965
Laboratory Mentor	Gerald A. Deneau, Ph.D.
Primary Research Theme at UM	Self-administration of drugs in monkeys

Post-Michigan Career	1965–1986	Instructor, Dept. of Pharmacology, The Jikei University School of Medicine
	1966–1976	Director, Dept. of Psychopharmacology, Preclinical Research Laboratories, Central Institute for Experimental Animals
	1976–1996	Director, Preclinical Research Laboratories, Central Institute for Experimental Animals

	1981–1986	Board Member, Central Institute for Animal Research
	1986–present	Adjunct Professor of Pharmacology, The Jikei University School of Medicine
	1997–present	Scientific Advisor, INA Research Inc.
Public Service	1970–1992	Member, Central Committee on Drug Affairs, Ministry of Health and Welfare
	1970–present	Board Member, Japanese Society of Clinical Pharmacology and Therapeutics
	1971–present	Board Member, Japanese Society of Neuropsychopharmacology
	1974–1998	Member, Scientific Advisory Panel on Drug Dependence, World Health Organization
	1974–1996	Board Member, Japanese Medical Society of Studies on Alcohol
	1975–1995	Board Member, Japanese Society of Toxicological Sciences
	1985–1994	Board Member, Japanese Pharmacological Society
	1985–1986	President, Japanese Society of Neuropsychopharmacology
	1988–1989	President, Japanese Society of Toxicological Sciences
	1992–1993	President, Japanese Society of Clinical Pharmacology and Therapeutics
	1994	Advisory Committee Member on Anti-drug Abuse Policy, United Nations Drug Control Program, Vienna
	1994–1997	President, Asian Society of Toxicology
	1995–1996	President, Japanese Medical Society of Studies on Alcohol
Honors	1994	Mochizuki Prize for Outstanding Achievement in Toxicology
Areas of Specialization		Drug dependence; clinical pharmacology (phase I); preclinical testing of drugs

Biographical Sketch

Fellow	Mitsuhiro Yoshioka, M.D., Ph.D.
Years at Michigan	1989–1990
Laboratory Mentor	Charles B. Smith, M.D., Ph.D.
Primary Research Theme at UM	Serotonin release in the CNS

Post-Michigan Career

1990–1991	Assistant Professor, Dept. of Pharmacology, Hokkaido University School of Medicine
1991–1997	Associate Professor, Dept. of Pharmacology, Hokkaido University School of Medicine
1997–present	Professor, Dept. of Pharmacology, Hokkaido University Graduate School of Medicine

Public Service

Member of the following societies:
> American Society for Pharmacology and Experimental Therapeutics (ASPET)
> Sigma Xi
> Japanese Pharmacological Society
> First Flutist and Manager of the Sapporo Symphony Orchestra

Areas of Specialization   Serotonergic nervous system pharmacology

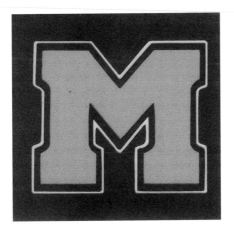

Appendix B1: Group Photographs of Early Beginnings and Michigan Reunions

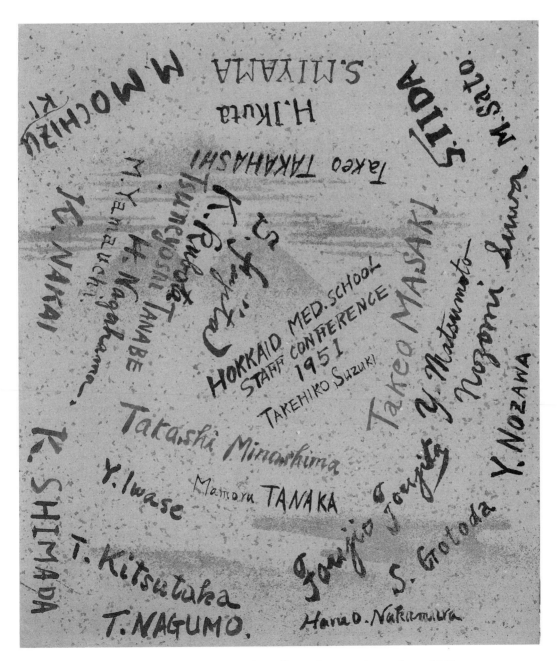

Hokkaido Medical School Staff Conference Attendees, 1951.

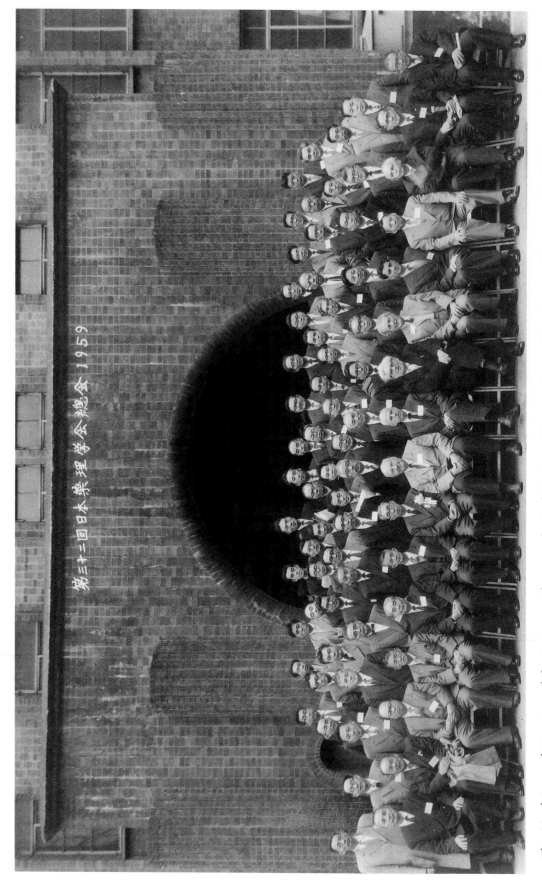

The 32nd Annual Meeting of the Japanese Pharmacological Society. The members of the Board of Trustees, Dr. H. Kumagai, President of the Society, Dr. M.H. Seevers, and other foreign guests are sitting in the middle of the front row. Tokyo, April, 1959.

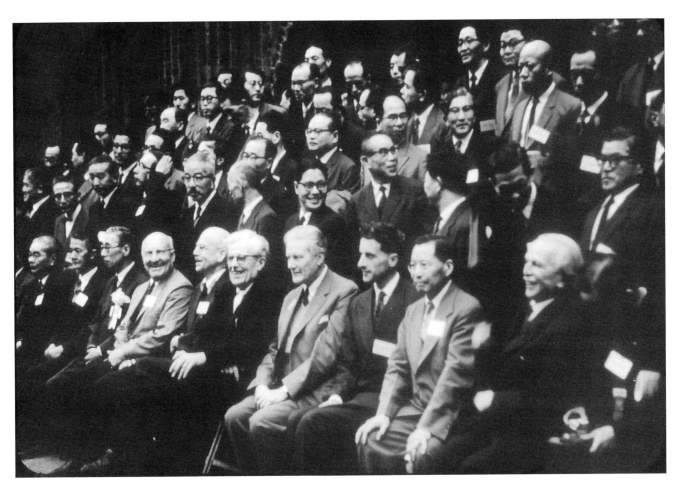

Japanese Pharmacological Society Congress in Tokyo, 1959.

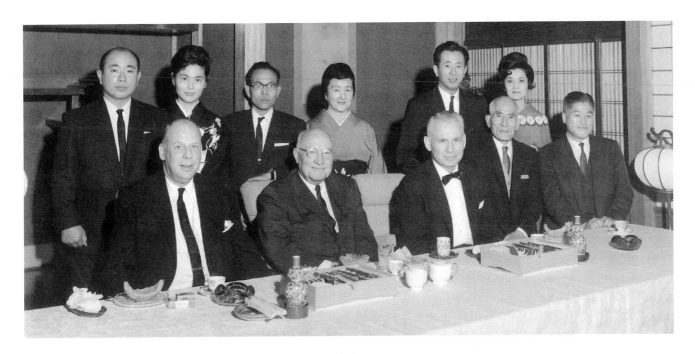

Meeting with foreign guests.

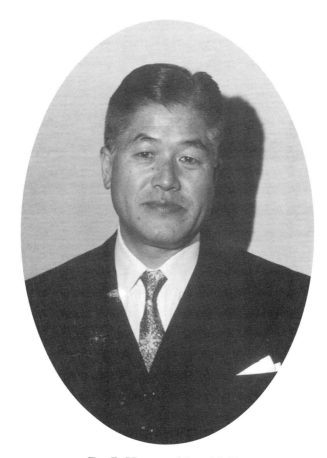

Dr. E. Hosoya, May, 1963.

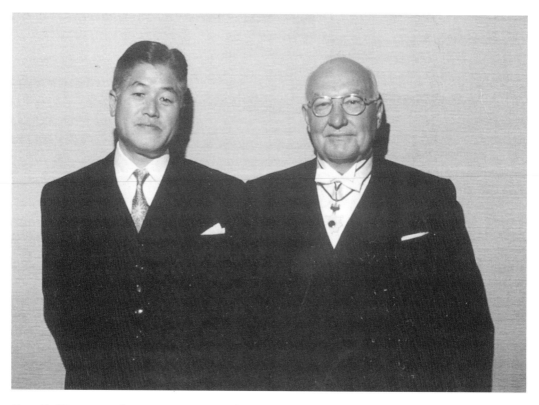

Drs. E. Hosoya and M.H. Seevers on the occasion of Dr. Seevers receiving the Order of the Rising Sun, Tokyo, May, 1963.

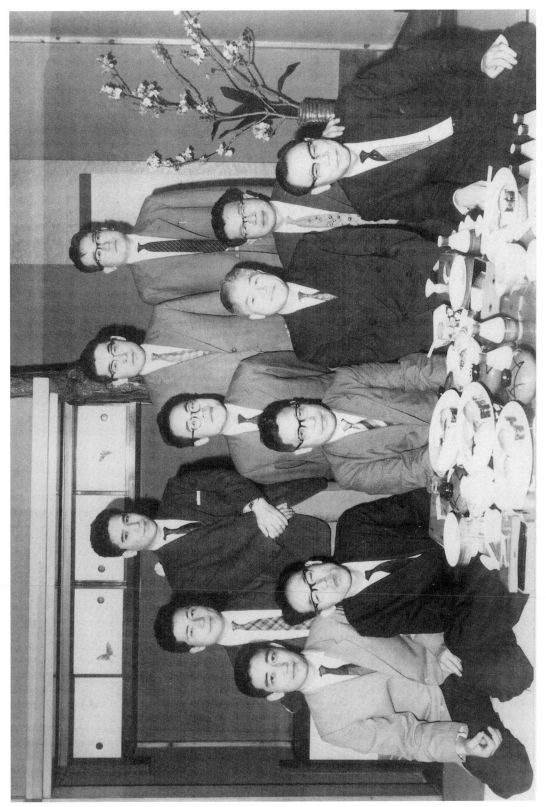

Michigan reunion in Tokyo, April 26, 1962.
Row 1 from left: Drs. A. Sakuma, Y. Ikeda, T. Tanabe, E. Hosoya, K. Shimamoto, Ohashi.
Row 2 from left: Drs. H. Kaneto, S. Ueki, K. Nakai, T. Akera, S. Takaori.

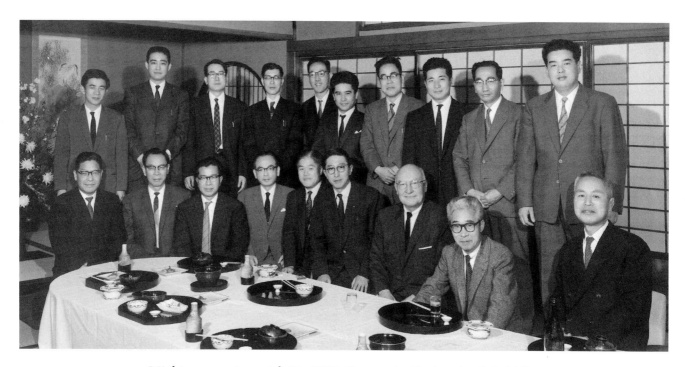

Michigan reunion with Dr. M.H. Seevers in Osaka, April 5, 1963.
Row 1 from left: Drs. T. Tanabe, Ohashi, K. Shimamoto, M. Yamasaki, E. Hosoya, I. Yamamoto, M.H. Seevers, H. Kumagai, Yamada.
Row 2 from left: Drs. R. Inoki, A. Sakuma, S. Takaori, N. Katsuda, Y. Ikeda, S. Ueki, K. Nakai, H. Kaneto, S. Hisada, K. Yamamoto.

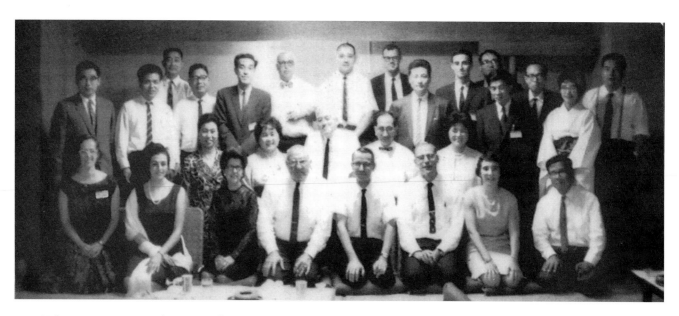

Michigan reunion at the XXIIIrd International Congress of Physiological Sciences in Tokyo, September, 1965. The guests include Dr. M.H. Seevers, Dr. and Mrs. F. Shideman, Dr. and Mrs. L. Woods, Dr. and Mrs. E. Domino, Dr. and Mrs. Pardo, and others.

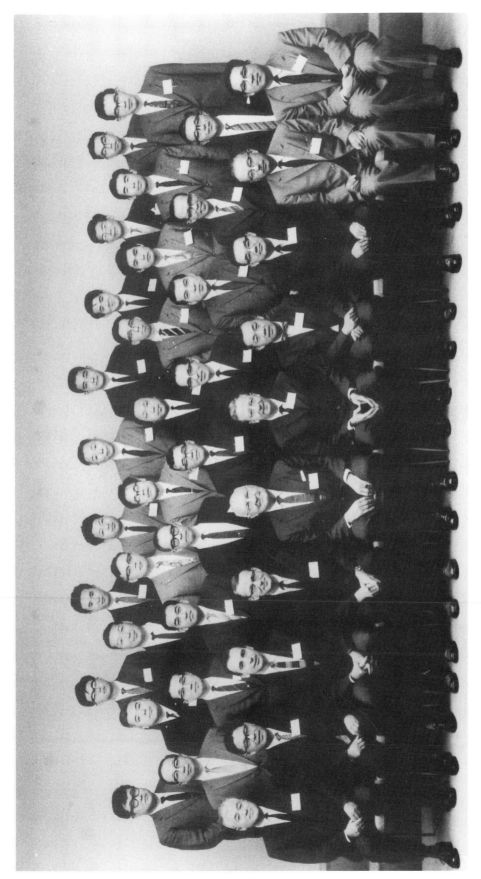

Conference on Clinical Pharmacology held in Sapporo as a satellite symposium of the XXIIIrd International Congress of Physiological Sciences in Tokyo, September 10, 1965.

Row 1 from left: Drs. E. Hosoya T. Tanabe, Demis, F.E. Shideman, M.H. Seevers, B. Uvnäs, L.E. Way, G.T. Okita, Takasugi, Hirai.

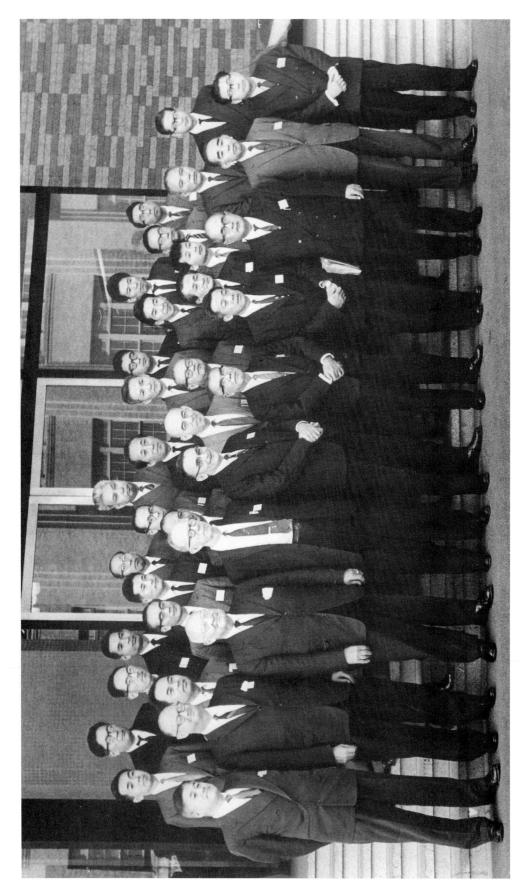

U.S.-Japan Joint Program Meeting on Narcotics held at the Ministry of Health and Welfare of Japan in Tokyo, October, 1965.
Drs. E. Hosoya, D. Cameron, M.H. Seevers, N. Eddy, H. Isbell, a Japanese minister, Drs. L.E. Way, A. Kasamatsu, A. Hayashi, H. Kono.
Row 2 from left: Government official, Dr. Ikagawa, unidentified official, Drs. H. Brill, T. Nakao, M. Kato, Haga, Government official, Government official.

Row 3 from left: Drs. H. Takagi, Y. Ikeda, H. Kaneto, S. Iida, T. Kobayashi, H. Utena, T. Ishikawa, Government official.
Row 4: Government official.

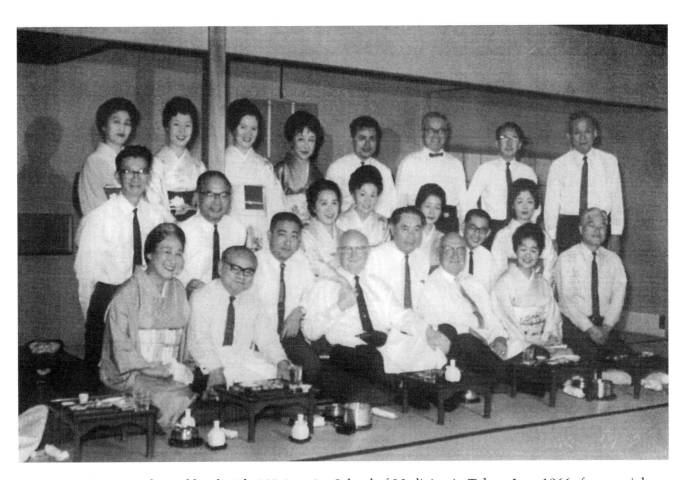

A reception party hosted by the Jikei University School of Medicine in Tokyo, June 1966 after special lectures by Dr. M.H. Seevers and Dr. F. Fraser from the USPHS, Addiction Research Center, Lexington, Kentucky.
Row 1 from left: Drs. T. Nakao, F. Fraser, M.H. Seevers, E. Hosoya.
Row 2 from left: Drs. Y. Omori, T. Tomii, A. Sakuma, K. Higuchi (President), T. Nomura.
Row 3 from left: Drs. T. Yanagita, R. Natori, T. Sakai, M. Matsuba.
All the ladies are hostesses.

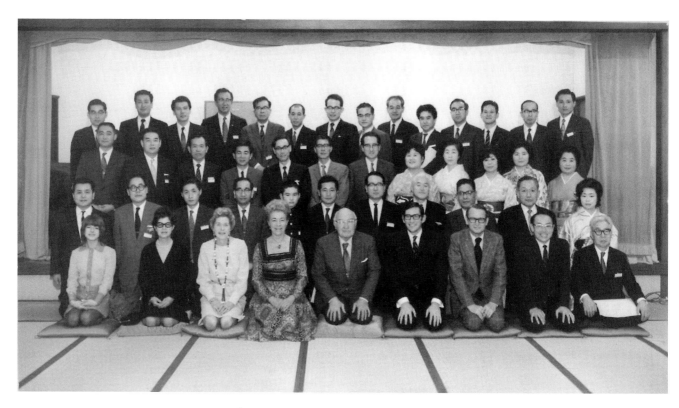

Michigan reunion in Tokyo, April 3, 1971.
Row 1 from left: Dr. Kumagai's daughter, Mrs. F. Shideman, Unidentified, Mrs. and Dr. M.H. Seevers, Unidentified, Drs. F. Shideman, Takemori, H. Kumagai.
Row 2 from left: Drs. T. Yanagita, K. Nakai, E. Hasegawa, S. Hisada, K. Yamamoto's son, Drs. H. Kaneto, S. Takaori, E. Hosoya, T. Tanabe, K. Matsuda, Unidentified.
Row 3 from left: Drs. A. Sakuma, K. Yamamoto, A. Tsujimoto, R. Inoki, S. Tadokoro, N. Katsuda, H. Ito, Mrs. Hosoya, Mrs. Ito, Mrs. Miyasaka, Mrs. Yanagita, Mrs. Kumagai.
Row 4 from left: Drs. T. Akera, I. Matsuoka, Y. Nakai, S. Hayao, K. Shimamoto, T. Iwami, T. Oka, M. Miyasaka, Y. Matsuzaki, S. Ueki, S. Miyata, T. Fukuda, S. Iida, M. Hitomi.

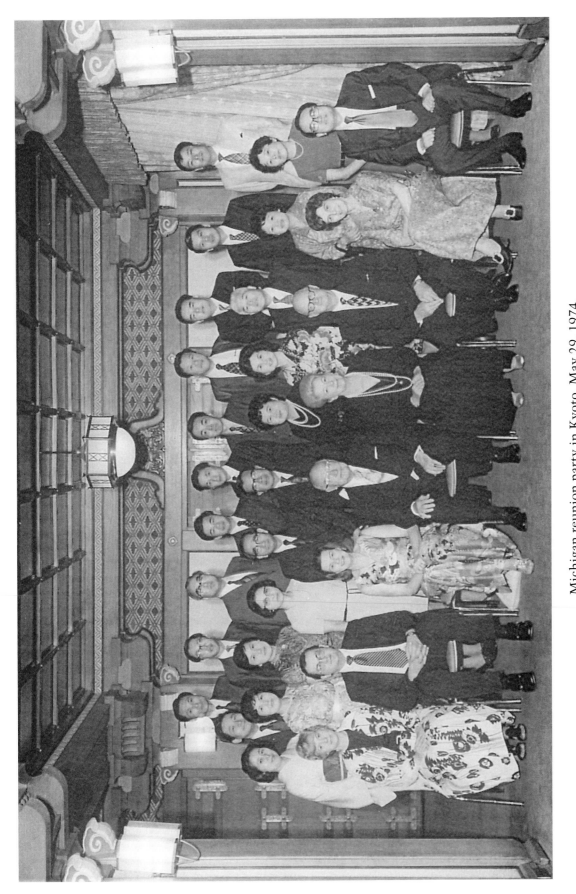

Michigan reunion party in Kyoto, May 29, 1974.
Row 1 from left: Mrs. and Dr. D. Jasinski, Mrs. D. Overbeck, Dr. M.H. and Mrs. Seevers, Dr. and Mrs. D. Cameron, Dr. S. Takaori.
Row 2 from left: Japanese wives, Drs. S. Hisada, K. Shimamoto, Japanese wives, Dr. E. Hosoya, Japanese wives.
Row 3 from left: Unidentified, Dr. M. Hitomi, Unidentified, Drs. S. Miyata, R. Inoki, E. Hasegawa, H. Takagi, M. Fujiwara, K. Yamamoto, Y. Nakai, I. Matsuoka.

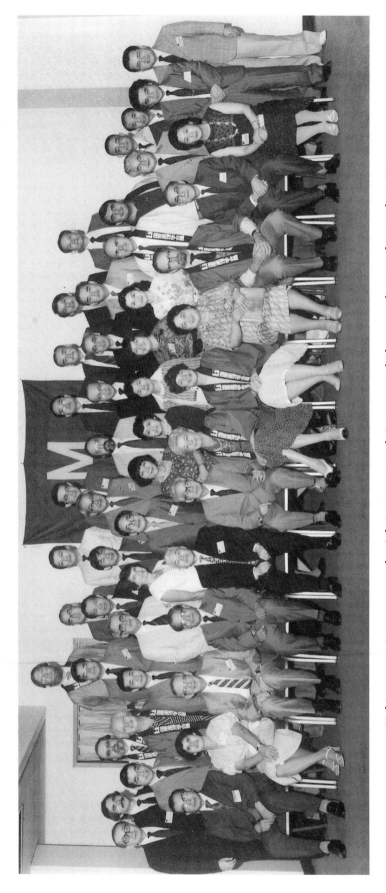

Michigan reunion party at the 8th International Congress of Pharmacology, Tokyo, July, 1981.

Row 1 from left: Dr. K. Shimamoto, Mrs. and Dr. T.M. Brody, Drs. T. Tanabe, E. Hosoya, H. Kumagai, Mrs. Seevers, Pam Seevers, Mrs. Hosoya, Dr. H. Swain, Dr. and Mrs. Murano.

Row 2 from left: Dr. T. Furukawa, T. Akera, J. Moore, H. Kaneto, Dr. and Mrs. H. Hardman, Dr. K. Nakai, Mrs. Miyasaka, Mrs. Iida, Mrs. Yanagita, Mrs. Gibbs, Mrs. Yamamoto, Drs. J. Gibbs, M. Miyasaka, Unidentified, Drs. S. Ueki, T. Yanagita.

Row 3 from left: Unidentified, Dr. J. McNeill, Unidentified, Drs. A. Tsujimoto, R. Inoki, Y. Matsuzaki, Unidentified, Drs. S. Iida, S. Tadokoro, K. Yamamoto, J. Woods, A. Sakuma.

Row 4 from left: Drs. J. Carney, S. Miyata, I. Matsuoka, T. Oka, S. Takaori, Unidentified, Drs. Y. Nakai, T. Fukuda.

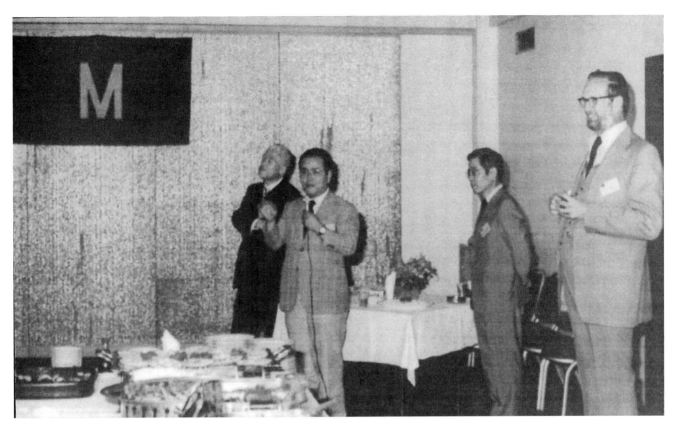

Michigan reunion party at the 8th International Congress of Pharmacology, Tokyo, July, 1981. From left: Drs. E. Hosoya, T. Yanagita, T. Akera, H. Swain.

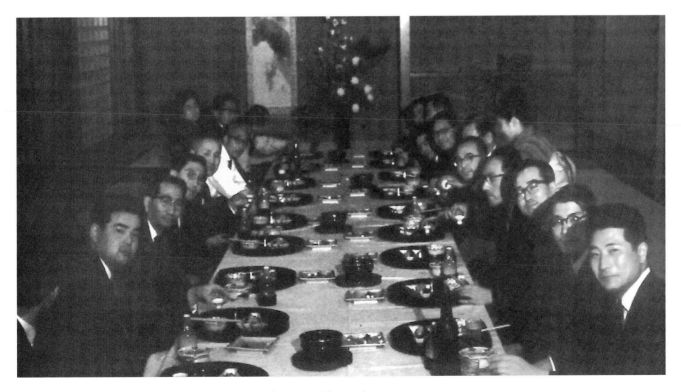

Michigan Fellows dinner party.

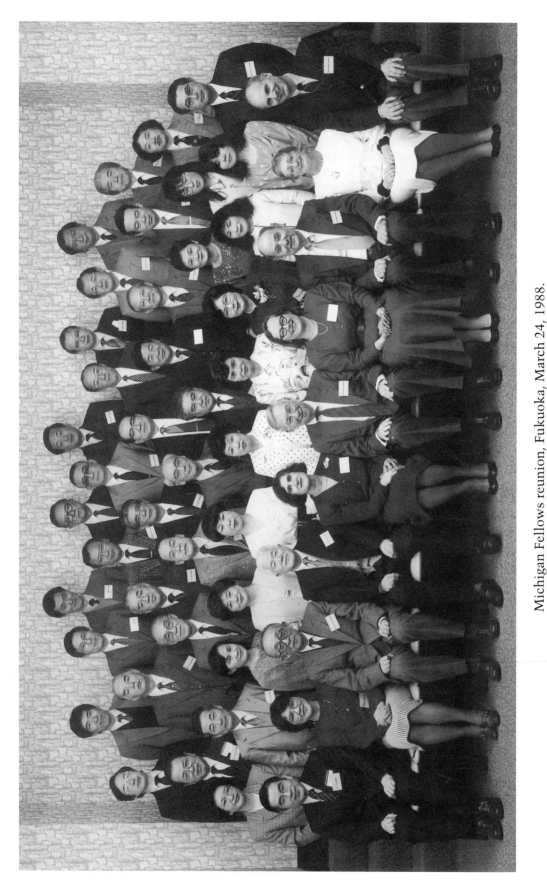

Michigan Fellows reunion, Fukuoka, March 24, 1988.

Row 1 from left: Drs. T. Akera, T. Furukawa, T. Furukawa, E. Hosoya, Mrs. and Dr. T. Brody, Mrs. and Dr. E. Domino, Mrs. and Dr. K. Moore.

Row 2 from left: Mrs. C. Akera, Dr. H. Kaneto, Mrs. Y. Katano, T. Ueki, E. Sakuma, T. Takaori, Y. Katsuda, T. Yanagita, Y. Yamada, E. Hori, Dr. K. Yamada.

Row 3 from left: Drs. T. Yanagita, T. Murano, K. Nakai, S. Tadokoro, S. Ueki, R. Inoki, Dr. Hanada, H. Yamada.

Row 4 from left: Drs. K. Takada, K. Yamamoto, S. Minamida, N. Katsuda, S. Takaori, T. Fukuda, T. Oka, T. Yamamoto.

Rows 5 and 6 from left: Drs. A. Uehara, H. Iwao, K. Temma, K. Takeda, S. Matsuoka, A. Sakuma, N. Fukuda, S. Yamamoto, M. Minami, T. Otani, T. Hirota, S. Matsumoto.

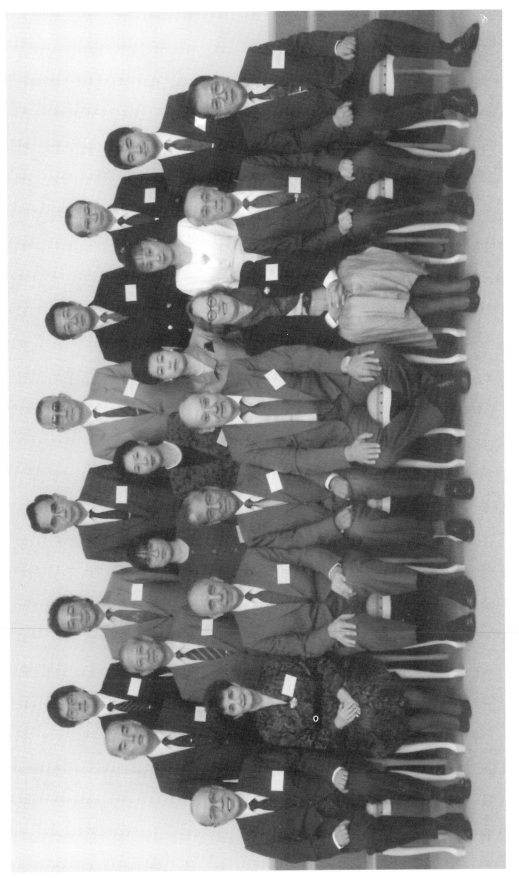

Michigan Fellows reunion and buffet, Sapporo, September 21, 1990.
Row 1 from left: Dr. S. Iida, Mrs. and Dr. B. Lucchesi, Dr. T. Tanabe, Dr. and Mrs. E. Domino, Drs. S. Tadokoro, T. Yanagita.
Row 2 from left: Drs. K. Yamamoto, T. Fukuda, Japanese wives, Dr. T. Endo.
Row 3 from left: Drs. M. Yoshioka, Monma, H. Saito, A. Sakuma, T. Otani, M. Minami.

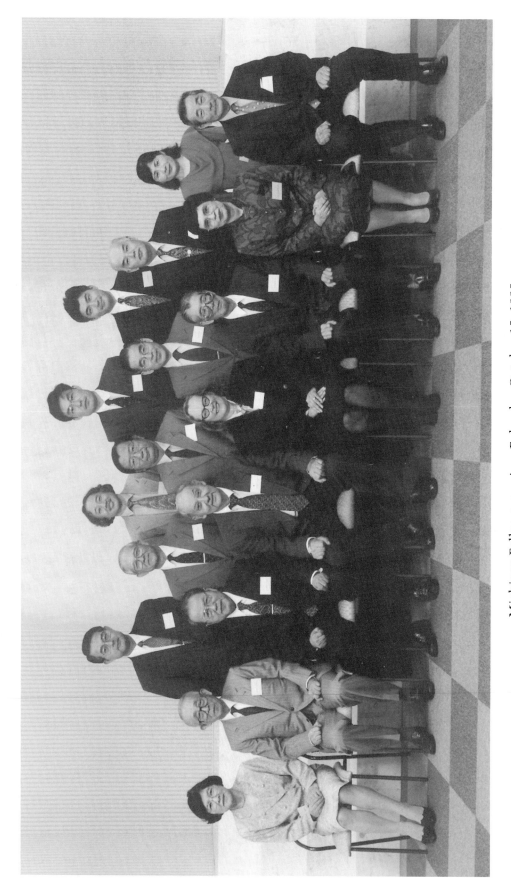

Michigan Fellows reunion, Fukuoka, October 15, 1995.
Row 1 from left: Mrs. and Dr. T. Furukawa, Dr. T. Yanagita, Dr. and Mrs. E. Domino, Dr. and Mrs. N. Katsuda, Dr. H. Kaneto.
Row 2 from left: Drs. K. Yamada, T. Fukuda, T. Hirota, T. Akera, K. Yamamoto, Mrs. Yamada.
Row 3 from left: Drs. T. Yamamoto, S. Iwata, T. Endo.

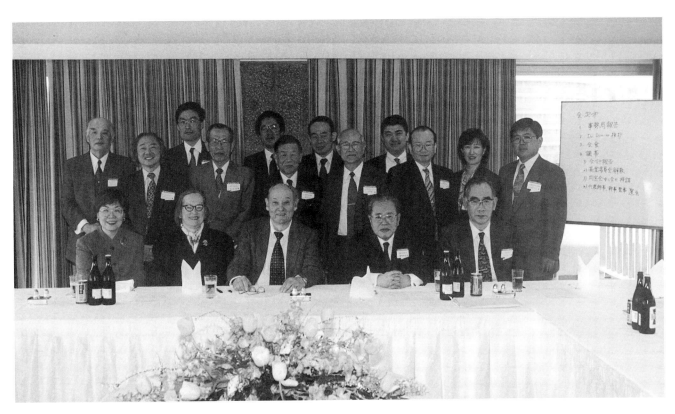

Michigan Fellows reunion at Kyoto International Congress Hall, March 24, 1998.
Row 1 from left: Dr. Y. Kohno, Mrs. and Dr. E.F. Domino, Drs. T. Yanagita, H. Saito.
Row 2 from left: Drs. K. Yamamoto, T. Yamamoto, A. Tsujimoto, R. Inoki, T. Fukuda, M. Minami,
H. Togashi, S. Kishioka.
Row 3 from left: Drs. S. Iwata, M. Yoshioka, T. Oka, T. Endo.

Appendix B2: Fellows and Guests Relaxing in Japan

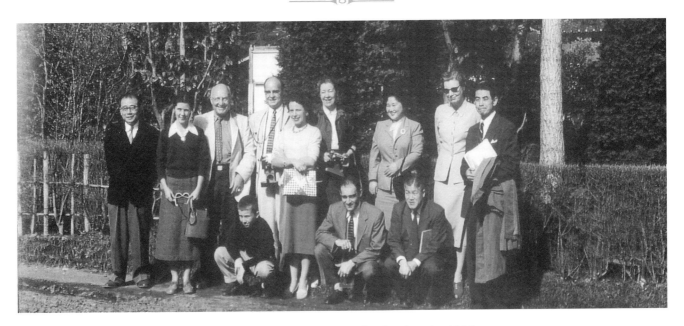

Near a bonsai garden north of Tokyo in 1956.

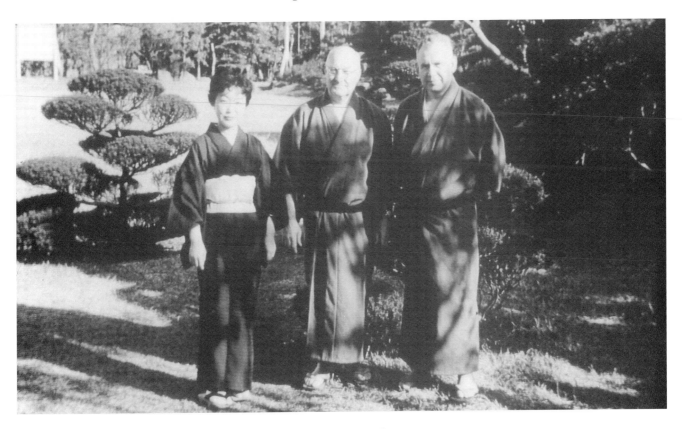

In Beppu, 1959.

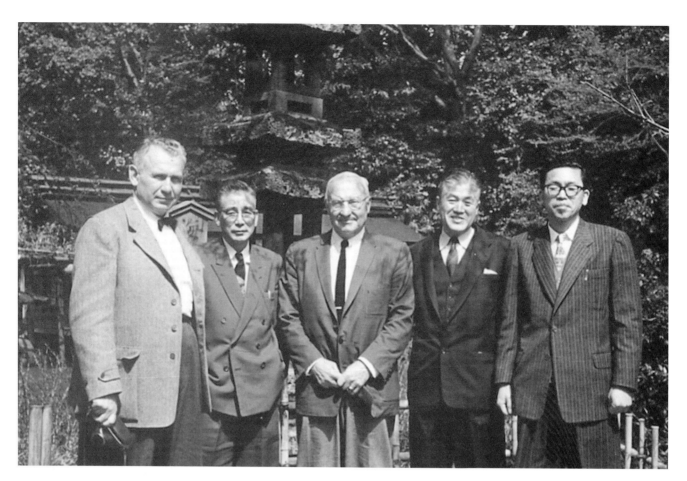

Drs. Compton, Seevers, Hosoya and friends in Japan, May, 1959.

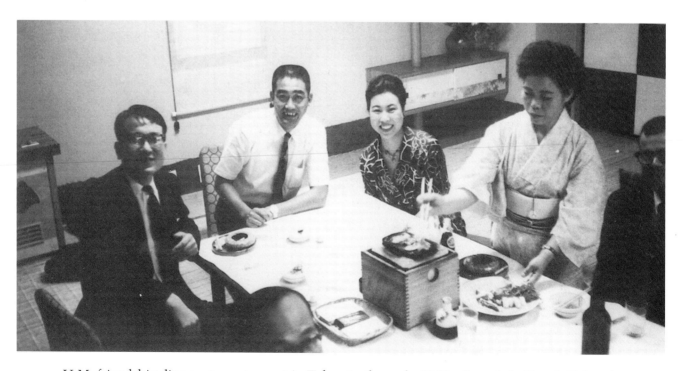

U.M. friendship dinner at a restaurant in Tokyo in the early 1960s. From left: Drs. S. Takaori,
Dr. and Mrs. A. Sakuma, hostess.

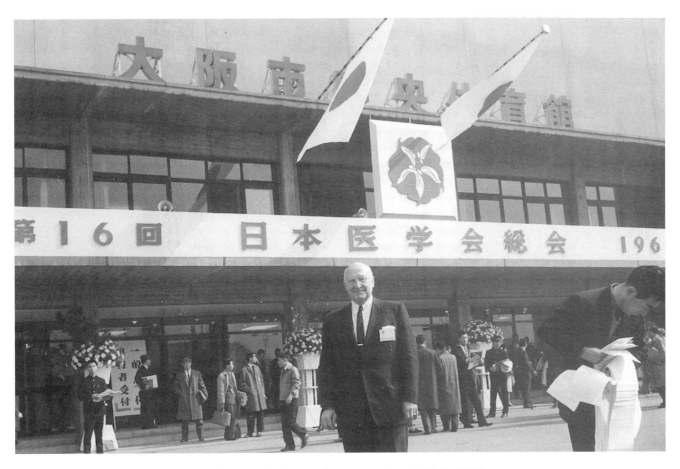

Dr. Seevers in front of a symposium hall in 1960.

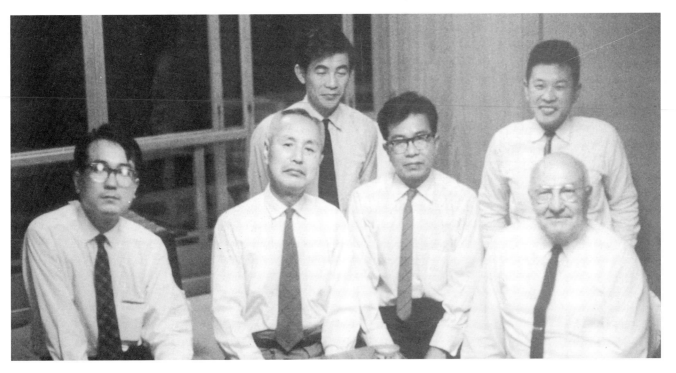

Michigan Fellows and friends with Dr. Seevers in Kyoto, May, 1963.
Row 1 from left: Drs. S. Takaori, Yamada, K. Shimamoto, M.H. Seevers.
Row 2 from left: Drs. R. Inoki, M. Fujiwara (aka Matsumura).

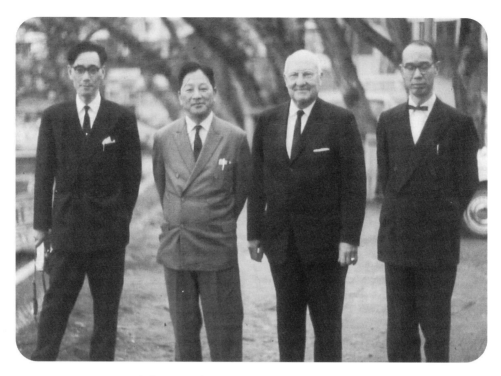

Dr. Tadokoro with Dr. Seevers and friends in 1964.

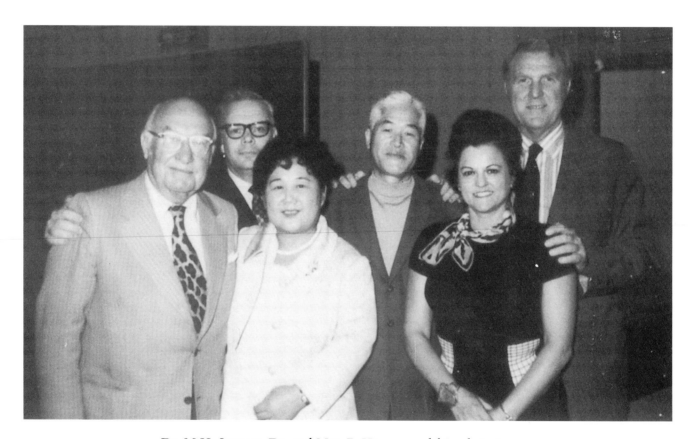

Dr. M.H. Seevers, Dr. and Mrs. E. Hosoya and friends in Japan.

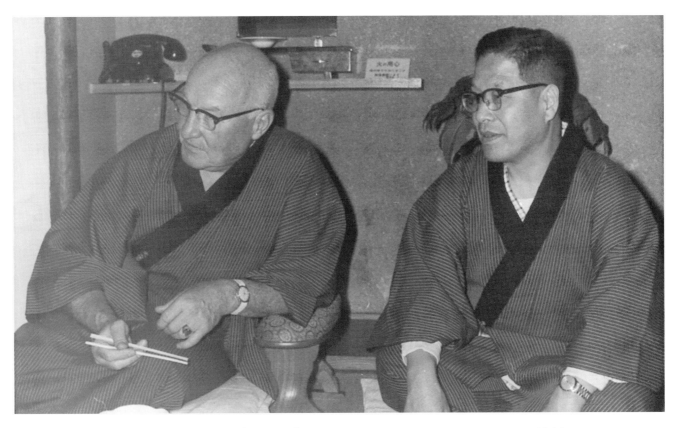

Drs. M.H. Seevers and T. Tanabe at a Japanese inn in Sapporo, August, 1966.

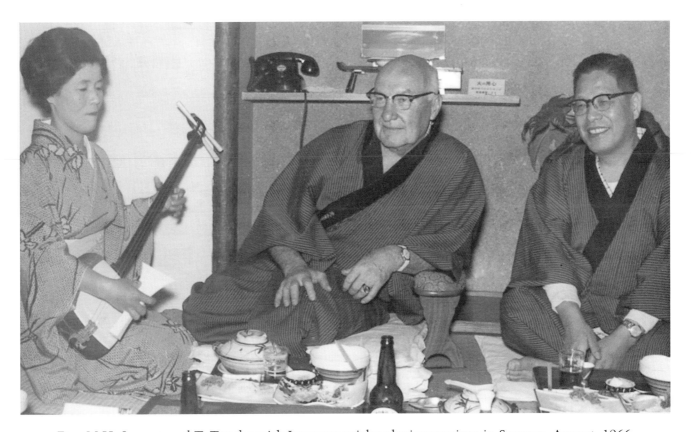

Drs. M.H. Seevers and T. Tanabe with Japanese geisha playing samisen in Sapporo, August, 1966.

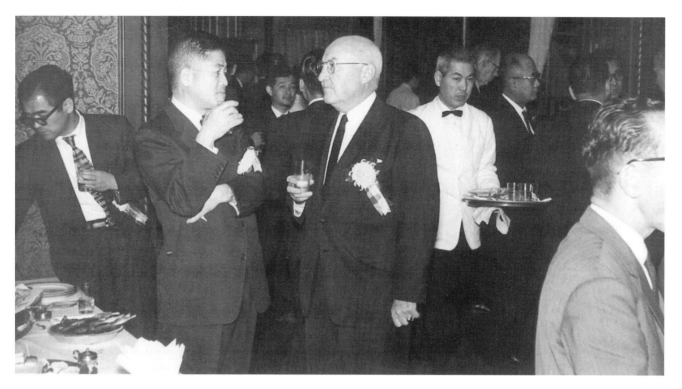

At a congratulatory party hosted by the Japanese Government following the ceremony to award Dr. M.H. Seevers the Second Class Order of the Sacred Treasure, Tokyo, 1967.

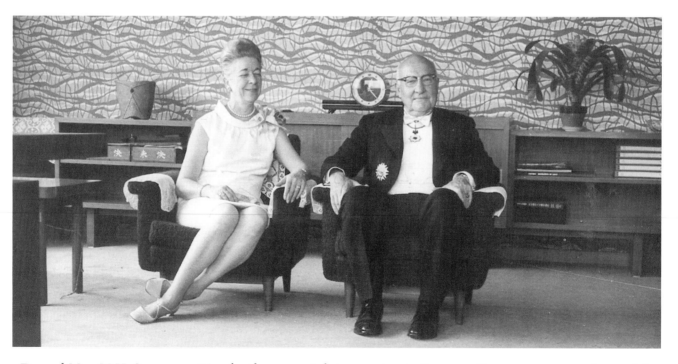

Dr. and Mrs. M.H. Seevers waiting for the congratulatory party at a Japanese Government guest house following ceremony to award Dr. Seevers the Second Class Order of the Sacred Treasure, Tokyo, 1967.

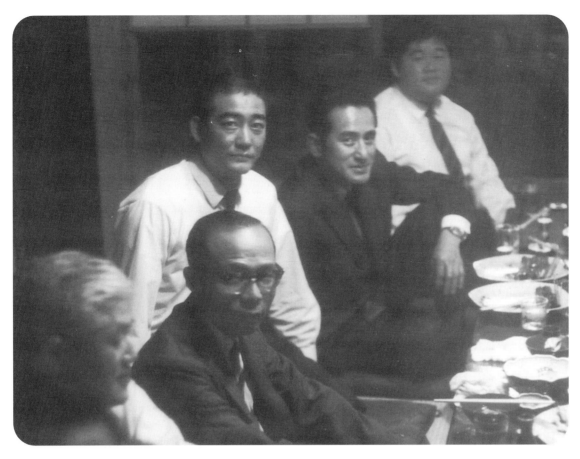

Eel party, 1966.

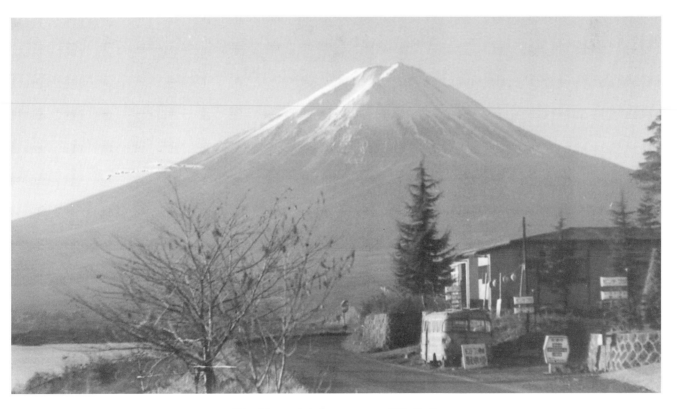

Dr. Matsuda's house near Mt. Fuji.

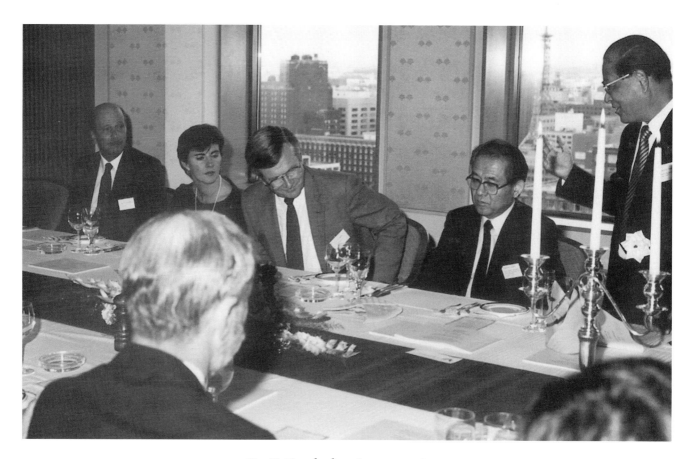

Dr. T. Tanabe hosting a meeting.

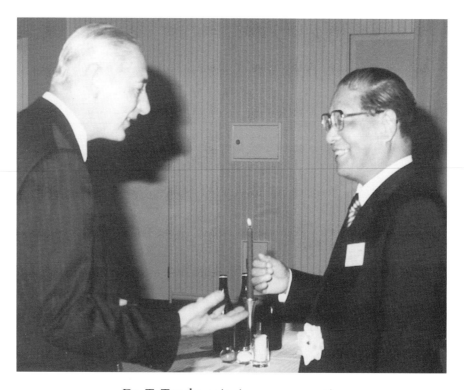

Dr. T. Tanabe enjoying a conversation.

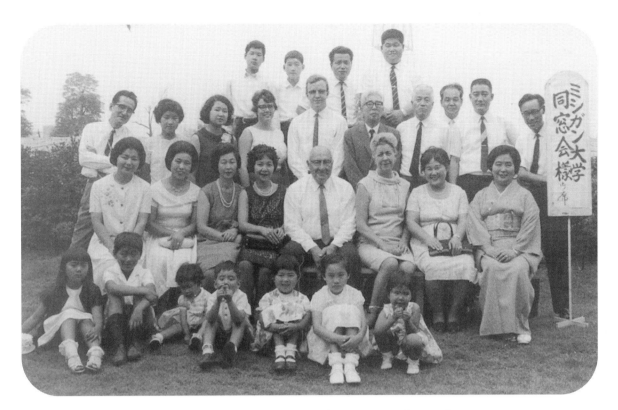

A Michigan family party at Hotel Otani in Tokyo, July, 1967.
Row 1. Children of Fellows.
Row 2 from left: Mrs. Yanagita, Mrs. Sakuma, Mrs. Ito, Mrs. Takokoro, Dr. and Mrs. M.H. Seevers, Mrs. Hosoya, Mrs. Kumagai.
Row 3 from left: Dr. H. Ito, 2 daughters of Dr. Ito, Mrs. and Dr. D. Dan, Drs. H. Kumagai, E. Hosoya, Y. Matsuzaki, A. Sakuma, S. Tadokoro.
Row 4 from left: 2 sons of Dr. Sakuma, Dr. T. Yanagita and a son.

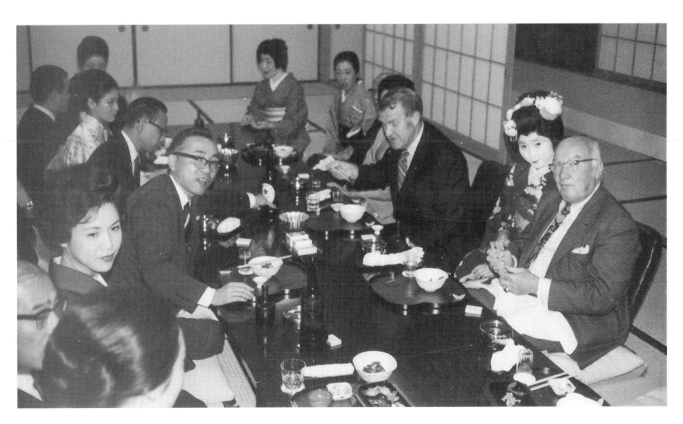

A Japanese party in 1971.

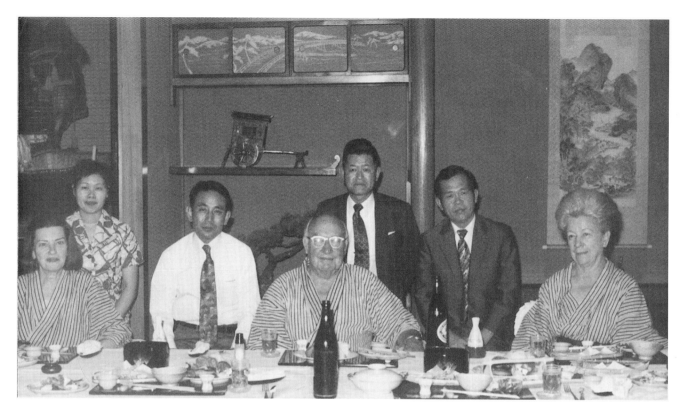

Dotty Overbeck, Dr. and Mrs. Seevers and friends at a Japanese dinner in Hiroshima, 1974.

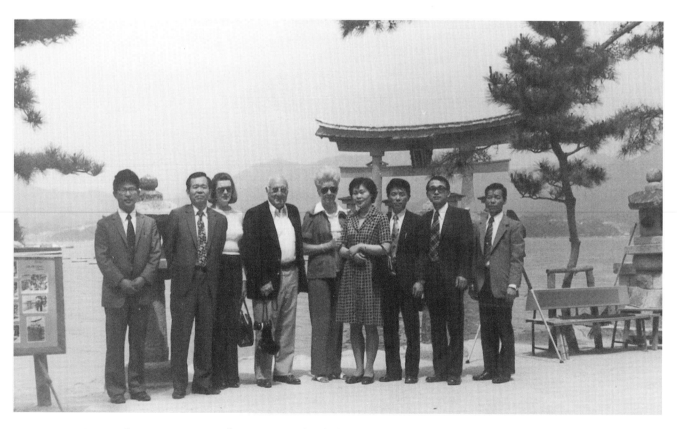

Dr. and Mrs. Seevers and Dotty Overbeck during one of the last visits to Japan, 1974.

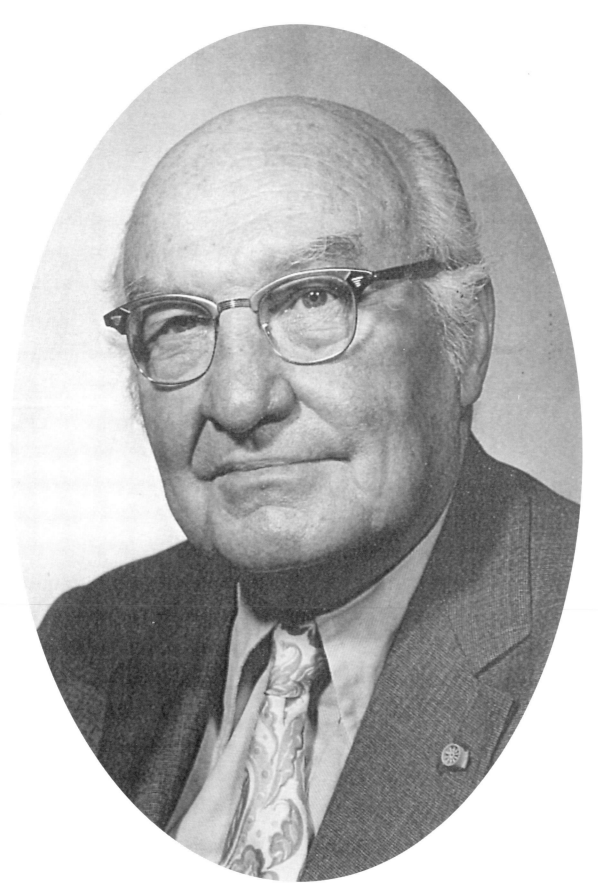

Dr. Seevers' portrait shortly before his death sent to Dr. T. Yanagita in Sheptember, 1997.

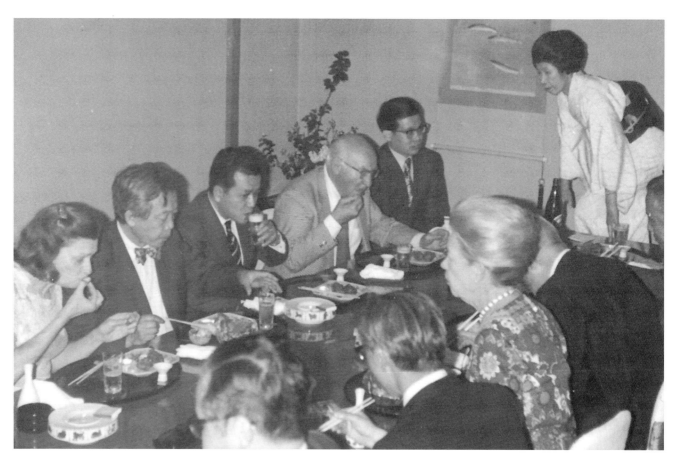

Dinner party in Japan.
Row facing camera: Dotty Overbeck, Drs. E. Way, T. Yanagita,M.H. Seevers, T. Oka.
Row with back to camera: Unidentified, Unidentified, Mrs. Seevers, Dr. E. Hosoya.

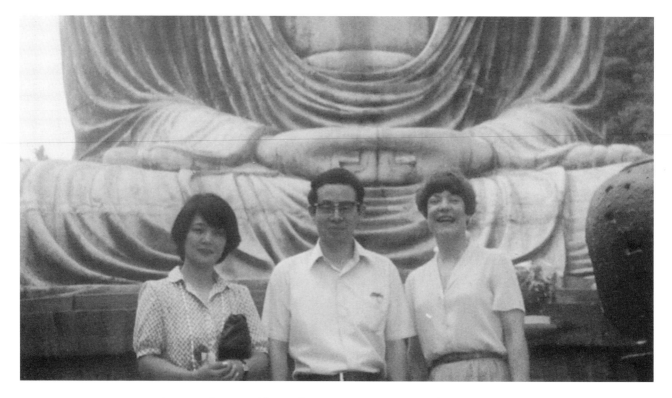

Mrs. and Dr. T. Oka and Pam Seevers in Kamakura, Japan.

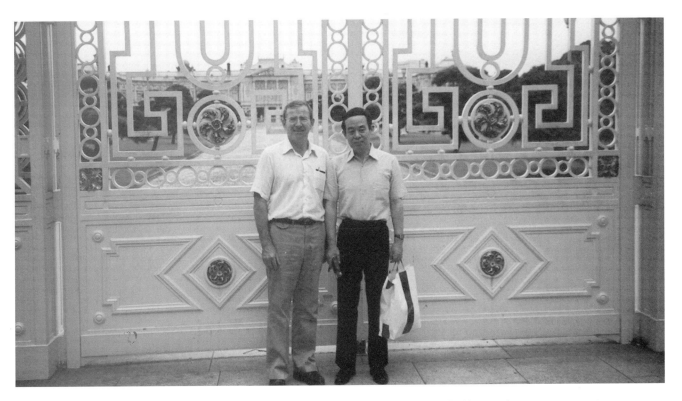

Drs. R. Ruddon and T. Oka in front of a reception hall in Tokyo.

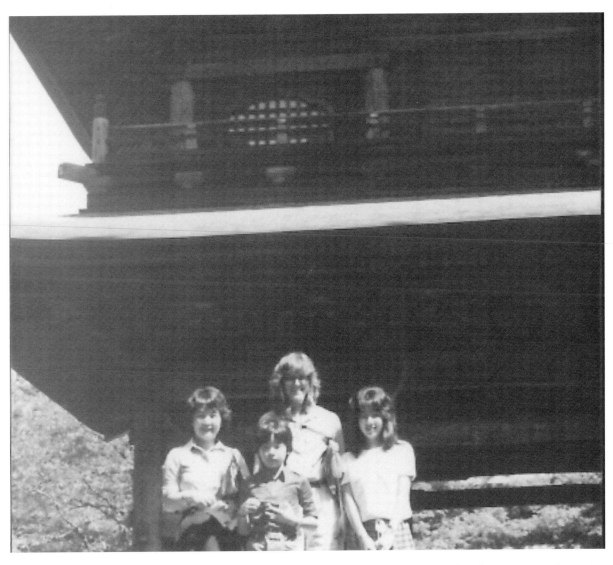

Mrs. Oka, son, Miss Kenner (undergraduate student in Dr. Oka's department), daughter at Kamakura, Japan.

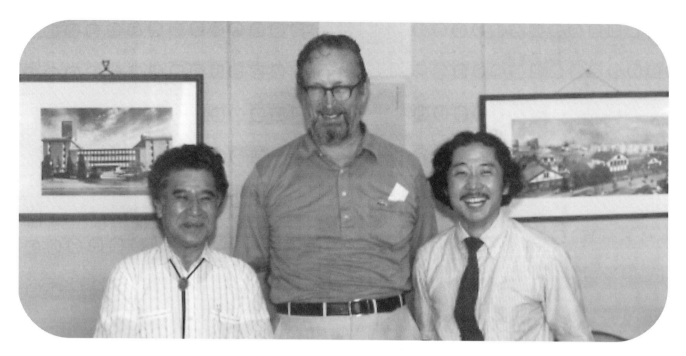

Drs. S. Ueki, H. Swain and T. Yamamoto in 1986.

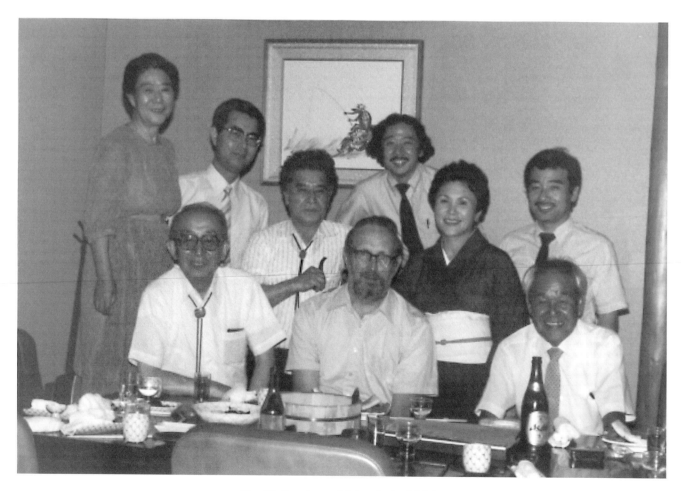

Dr. H. Swain and friends in 1986.

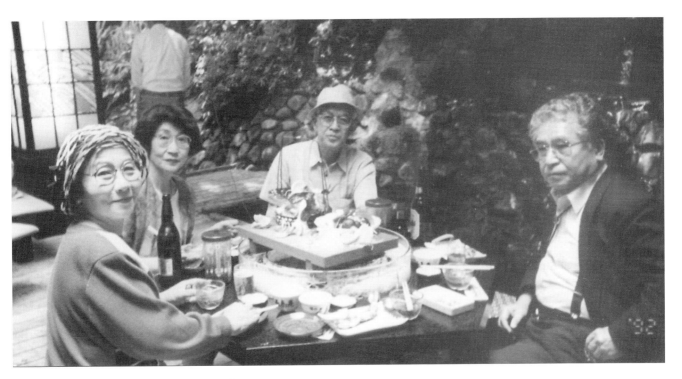

Dr. and Mrs. S. Ueki and friends in 1992.

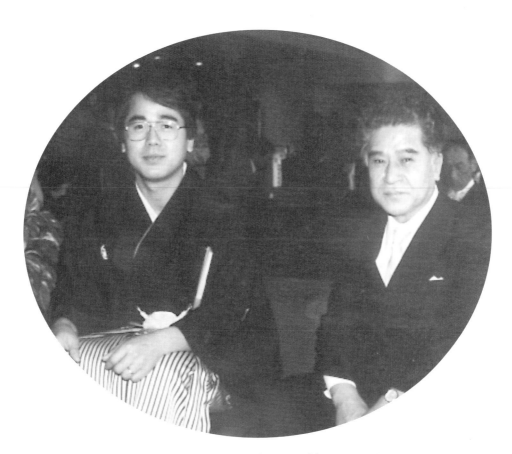

Dr. S. Ueki dressed up for a wedding reception.

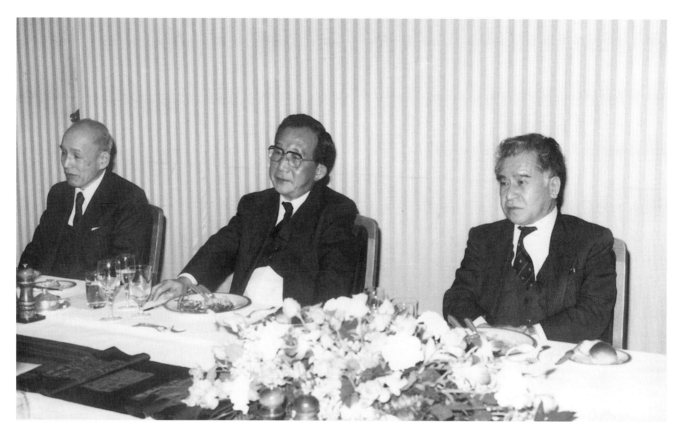

Dr. S. Ueki at a luncheon meeting with colleagues.

Appendix B3. Fellows and Colleagues in the United States and Their Return to Japan

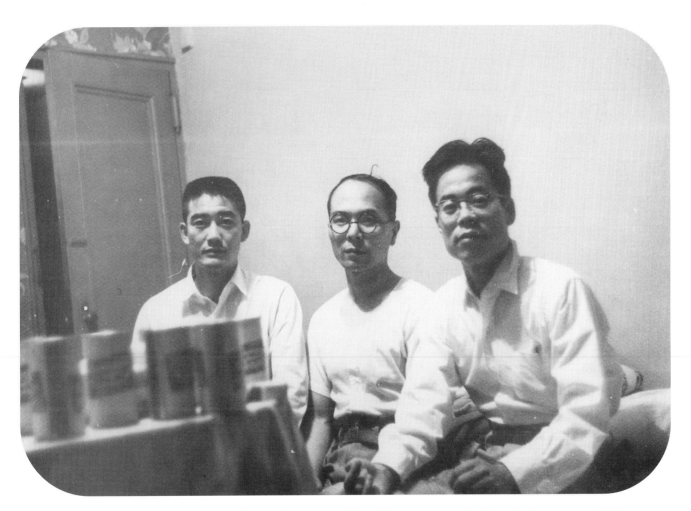

Drs. A. Sakuma, S. Ebashi, and K. Nakai in Dr. Ebashi's apartment in New York, August, 1959.

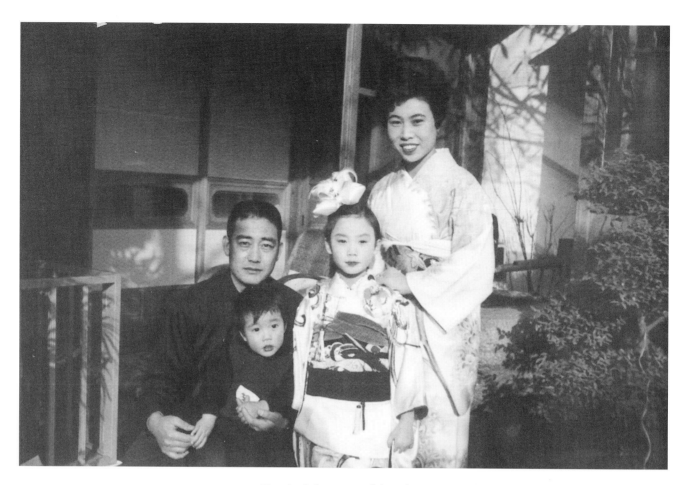

Dr. A. Sakuma and family.

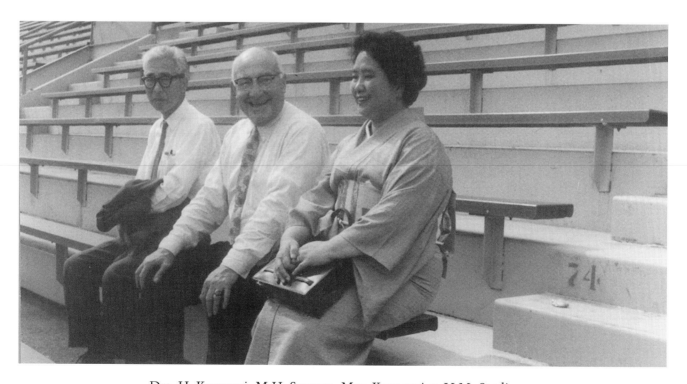

Drs. H. Kumagai, M.H. Seevers, Mrs. Kumagai at U.M. Stadium.

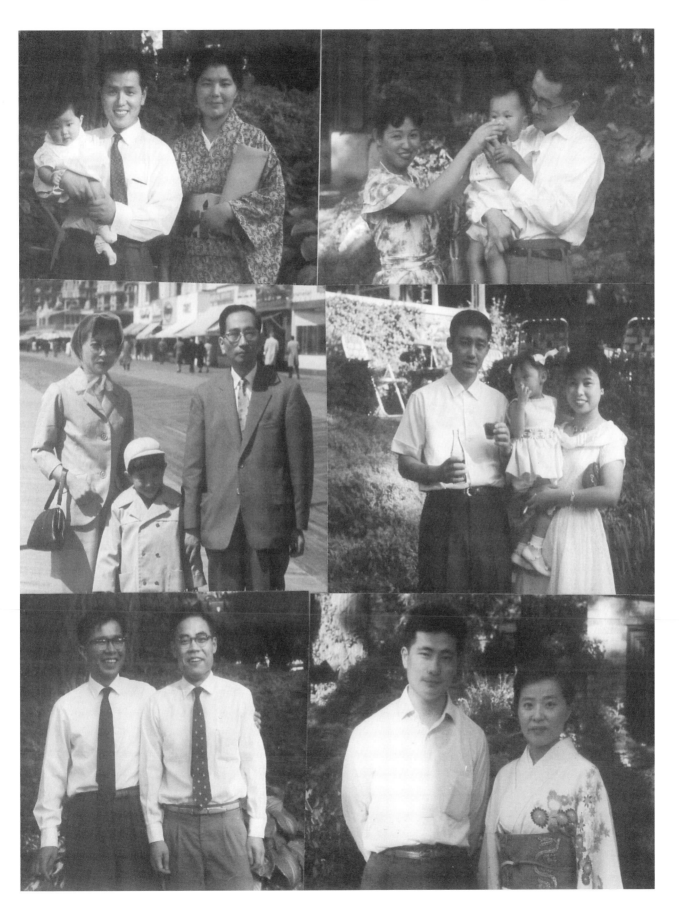

Some Michigan Fellows and families in 1961.

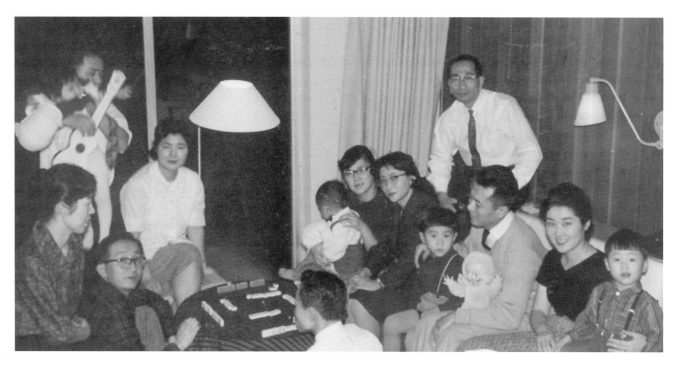

Christmas party of Japanese families in Ann Arbor, December, 1961.

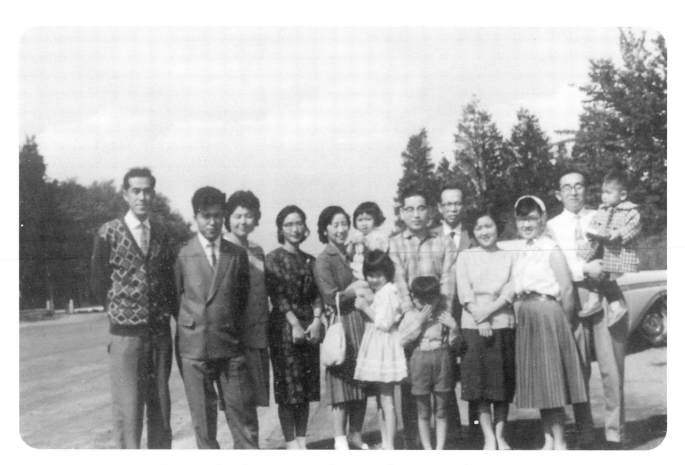

Japanese families at Point Pelee, Canada in September, 1962.

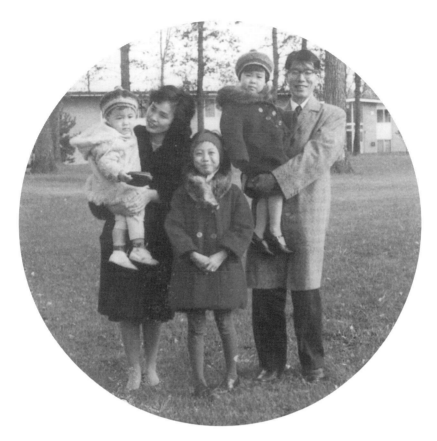

Dr. Katsuda and family in 1965.

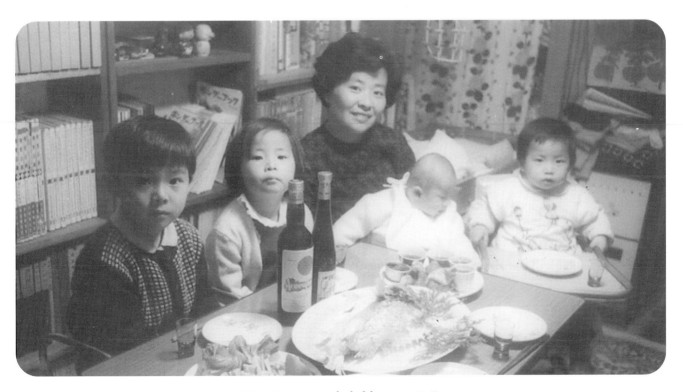

Mrs. Kaneto and children in 1967.

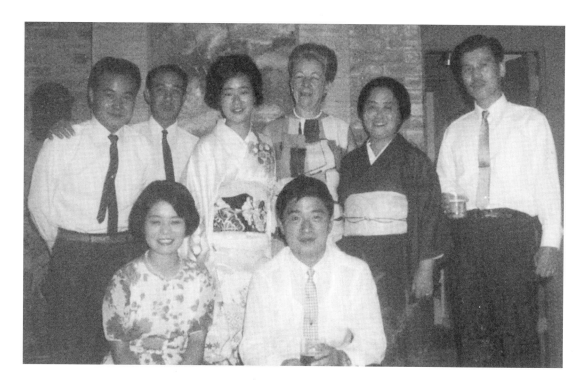

A party with Mrs. Seevers in 1966.

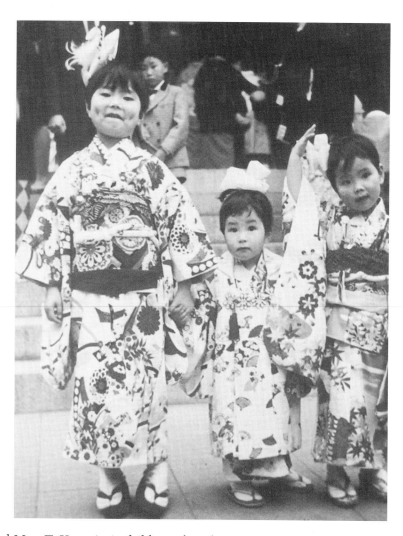

Dr. and Mrs. T. Yanagita's children after their return to Japan, November, 1966.

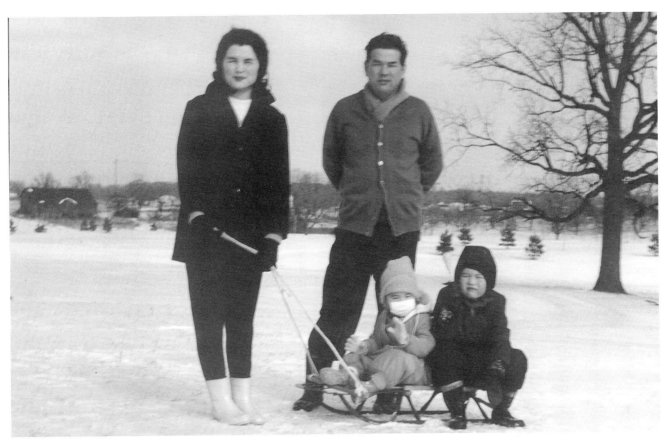

Dr. K. Yamamoto and family on the frozen Huron River, Ann Arbor, Michigan, January, 1965.

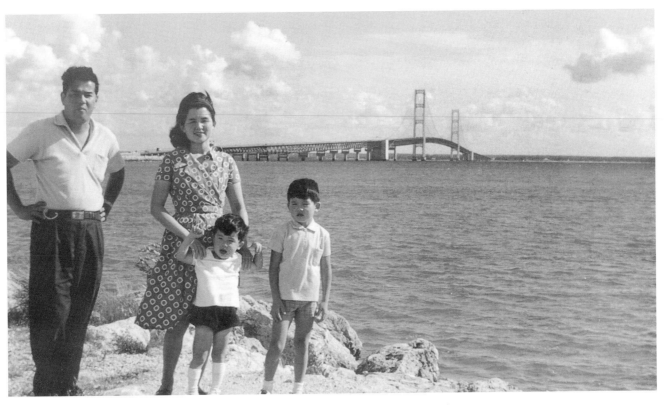

Dr. K. Yamamoto and family at the Mackinac Bridge connecting the lower and upper peninsulas of Michigan, August, 1964.

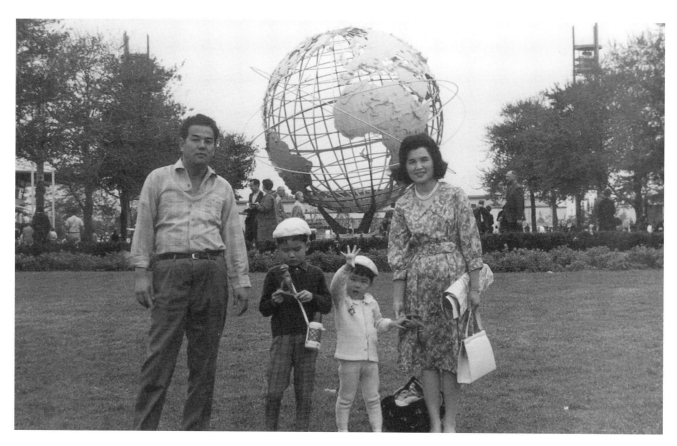

Dr. K. Yamamoto and family at the World's Fair in Queens, New York, summer, 1964.

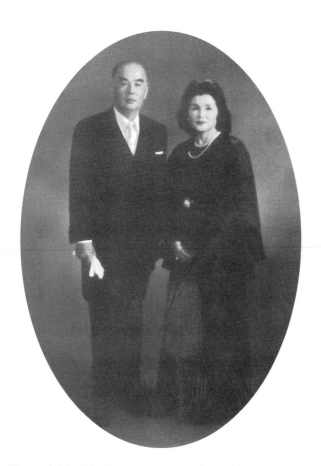

Dr. and Mrs. K. Yamamoto's 30th anniversary, November 27, 1988.

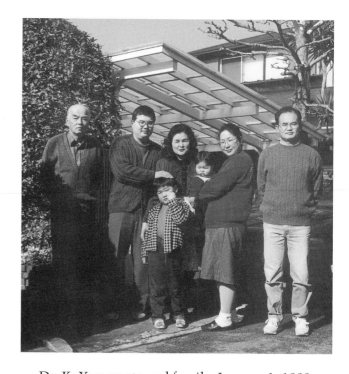

Dr. K. Yamamoto and family, January 1, 1998.

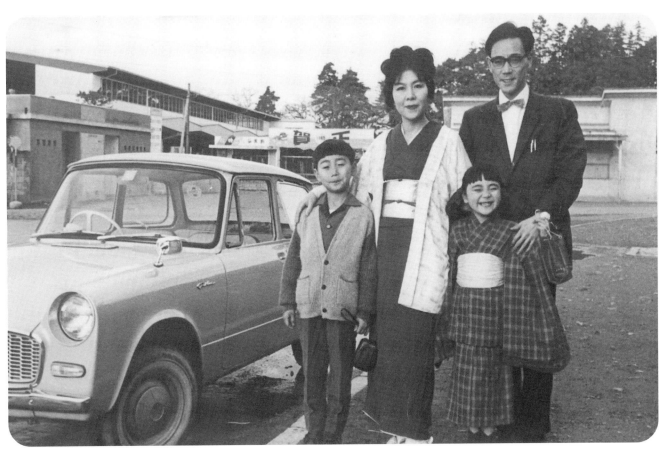

Dr. and Mrs. Tadokoro and children returning to Japan after 1967.

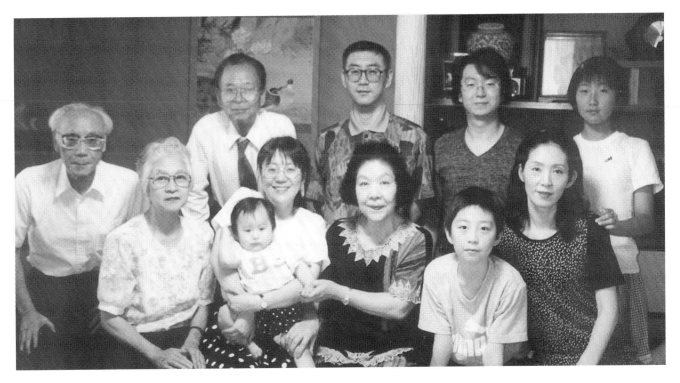

Dr. S. Tadokoro and family in July, 1998.

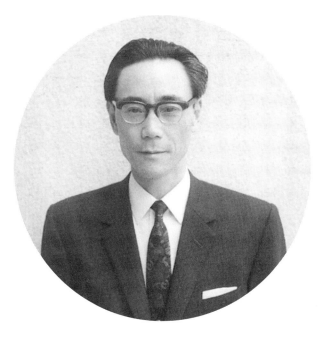

Dr. S. Tadokoro while at the University of Michigan in 1965.

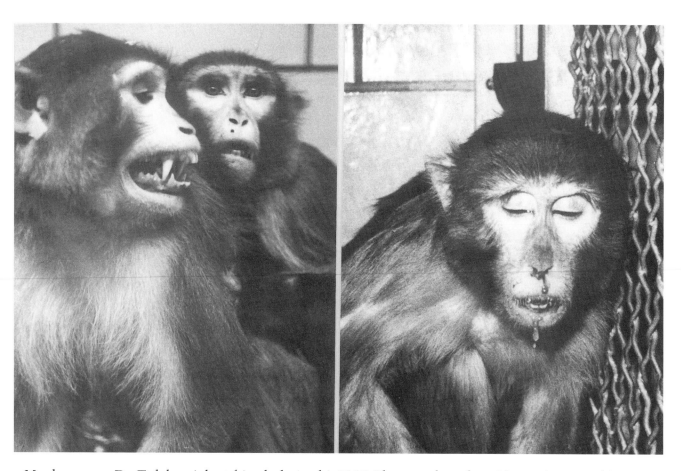

Monkeys were Dr. Tadokoro's best friends during his U.M. Pharmacology days. He was interested in morphine-dependent monkeys. The pictures show withdrawal signs of morphine-dependent monkeys. The one on the left foreground is the boss and was quite dangerous, especially during withdrawal.

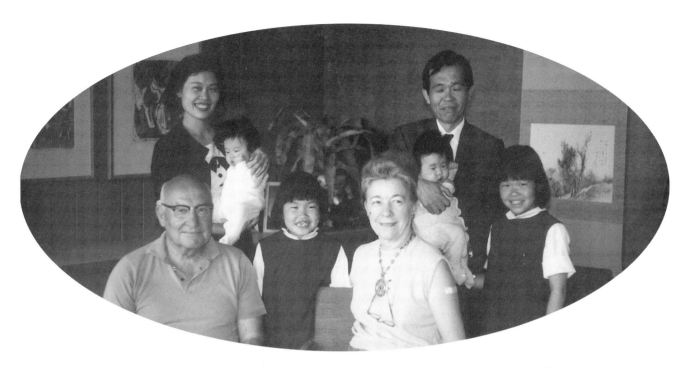

Dr. A. Tsujimoto and family with Dr. and Mrs. Seevers while in Ann Arbor.

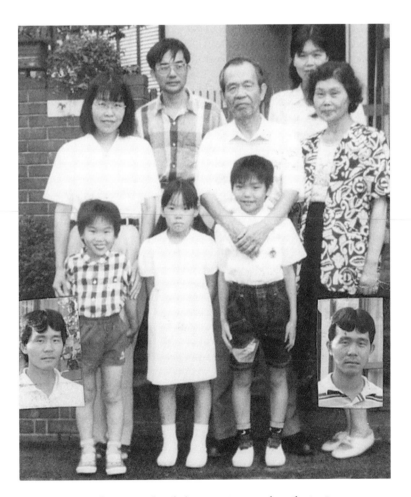

Recent photograph of the Tsujimoto family in Japan,
September 13, 1998.

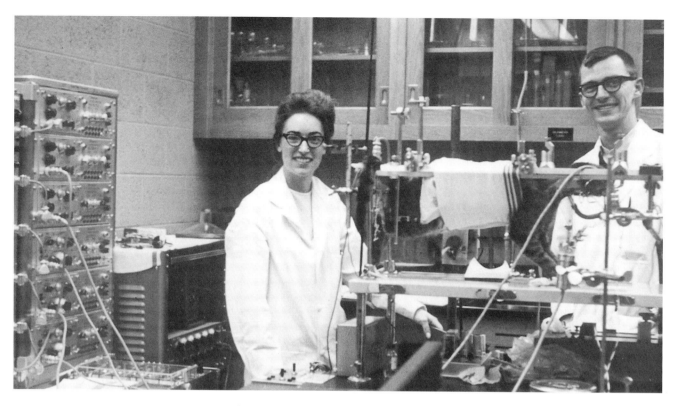

Lab photo taken by Dr. A. Tsujimoto during his stay in Ann Arbor.

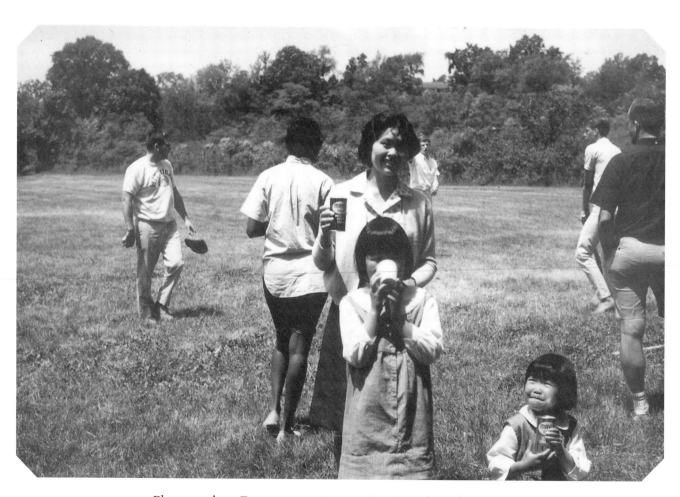

Pharmacology Department picnic at Dr. Towsley's farm, 1966.

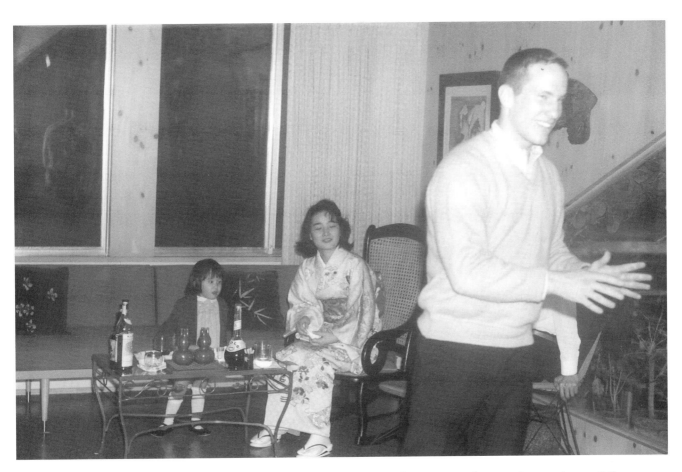

Party at Dr. Seevers' home. Left to right — Dr. Oka's daughter, Mrs. Oka, Dr. Seevers' son, Giles.

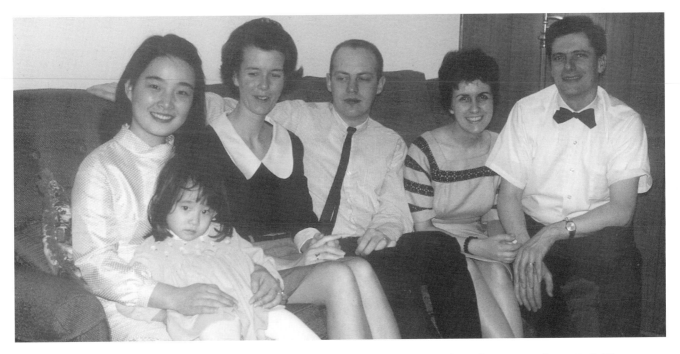

Party at Dr. C.C. Hug's home. Left to right — Mrs. Oka, daughter, friends, Mrs. and Dr. C.C. Hug.

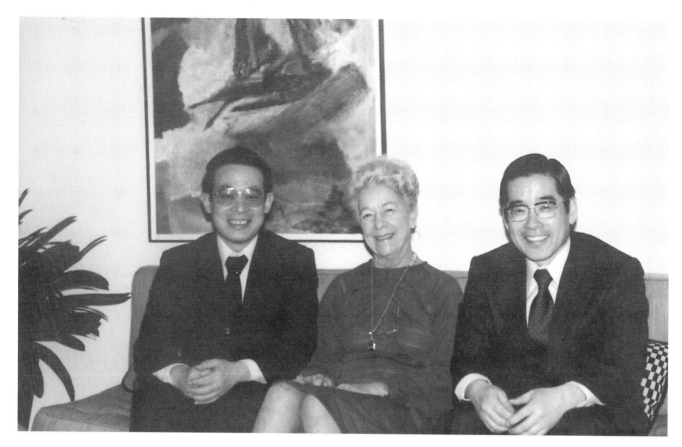

At Mrs. Seevers' home. Left to right — Dr. Oka, Mrs. Seevers, Dr. Akera.

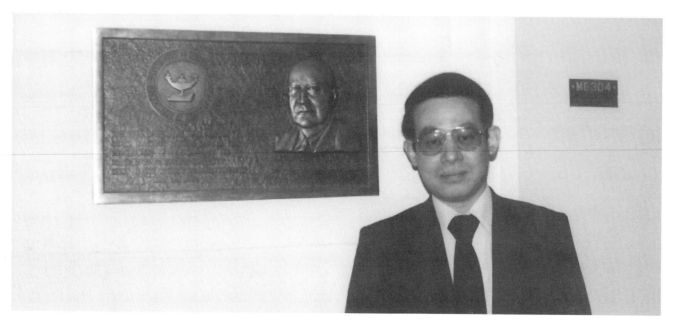

Dr. Oka at the U.M. Pharmacology Centennial celebration with Seevers' memorial plaque in background.

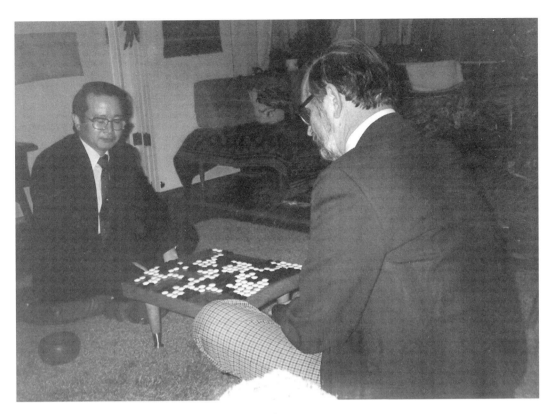

Who is winning?

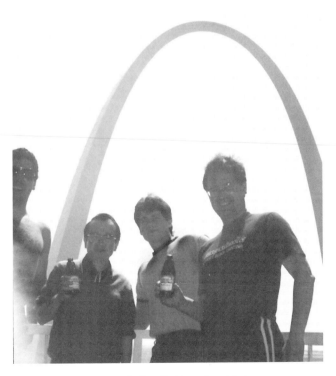

Dr. M. Minami with Dr. B. Lucchesi laboratory personnel in front of the Gateway Arch at 1986 FASEB meeting in St. Louis, Missouri.
Left to right: T. Pope, Dr. M. Minami,
M. Gallas. E. Driscoll.

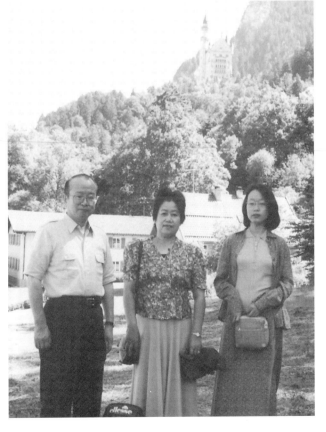

Dr. and Mrs. M. Minami and daughter, 1998.

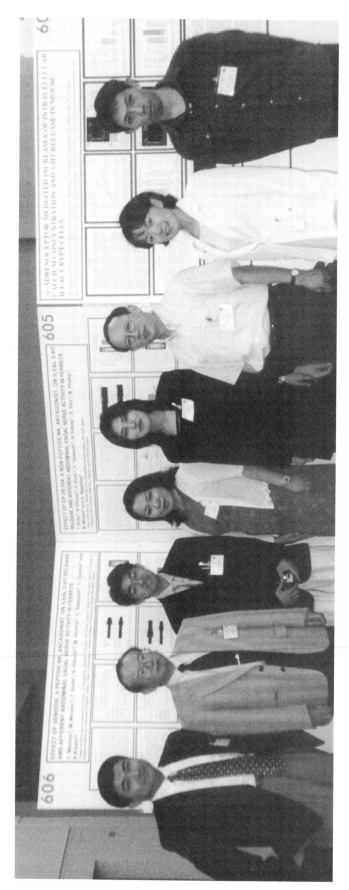

Dr. M. Minami and staff at the IUPHAR meeting in Munich, 1998.

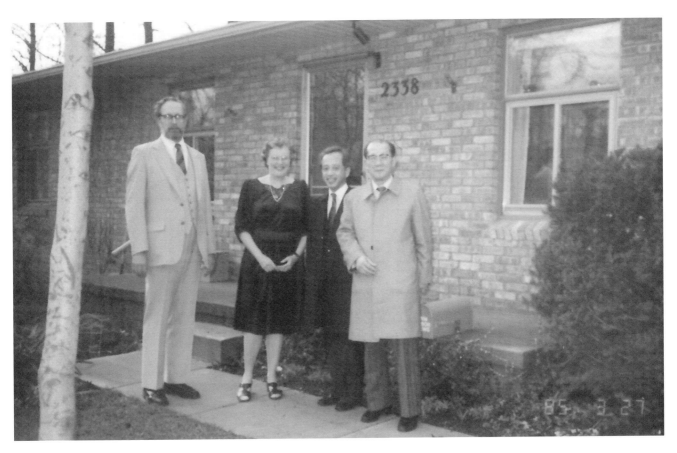

Outside of Dr. H. Swain's house in Ann Arbor, March 27, 1985.

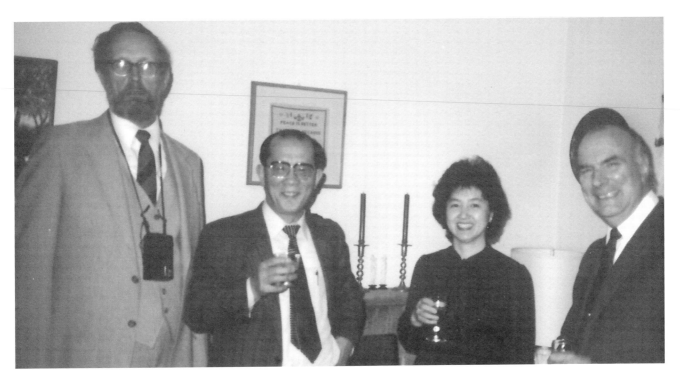

Enjoying a party at Dr. H. Swain's house, March 27, 1985.

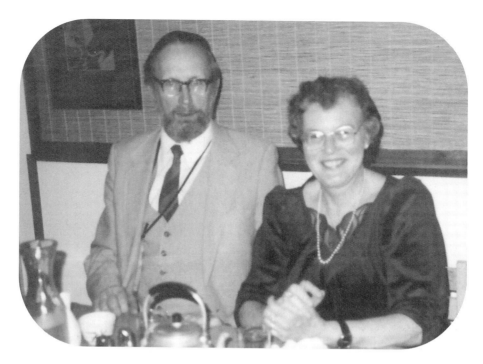

Henry and Vicki Swain hosting a dinner, March 27, 1985.

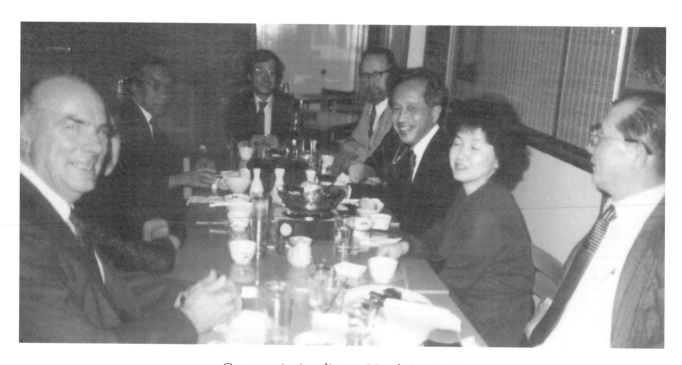

Guests enjoying dinner, March 27, 1985.

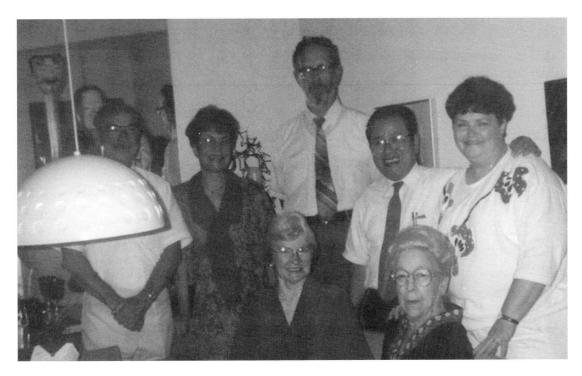

At Mrs. Seevers' apartment in Ann Arbor, June, 1989.
Left to right — Pam Seevers' friend, Pam Seevers, Dr. H. Swain, Mrs. McCarthy, Dr. T. Yanagita, Mrs. Seevers, household helper.

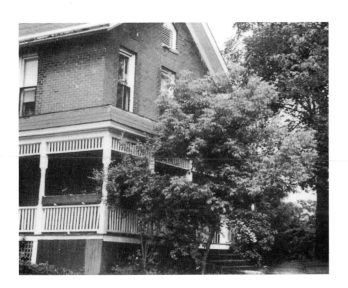

The house on High Street, Ann Arbor.

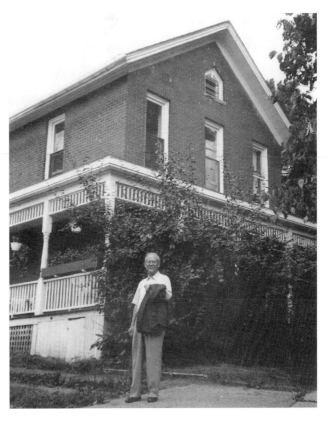

Dr. T. Fukuda revisiting the house on High Street, Ann Arbor, 1994.

Appendix B4. Faculty and Fellows of University of Michigan Department of Pharmacology and Friends

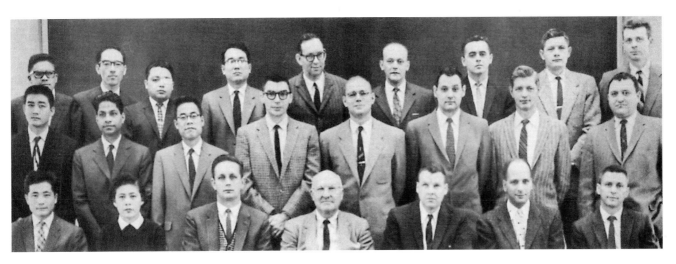

Department of Pharmacology, University of Michigan, 1960.
Row 1 from left: Drs. H. Kaneto, P. Bukhamana, H. Swain, M. Seevers, E. Carr, Jr., E. Cafruny, L. Beck.
Row 2 from left: Drs. A. Sakuma, A. Misra, K. Nakai, W. Baird, L. Woods, E. Domino, D. Knapp, L. Mellett.
Row 3 from left: Drs. G. Alcantara, Y. Ikeda, H. Vasquez, S. Takaori, T. Brody, A. Aste, H. Hardman, D. Bennett, G. Deneau.

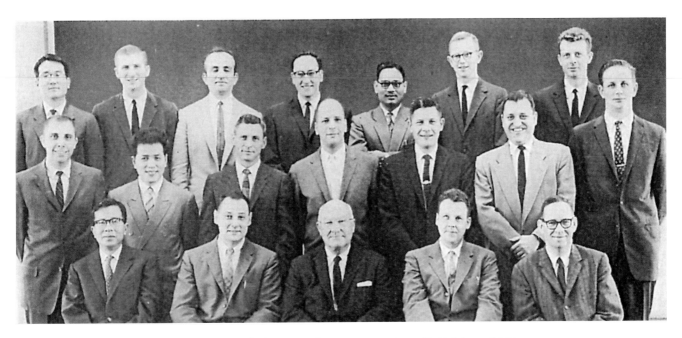

Department of Pharmacology, University of Michigan 1961.
Row 1 from left: Drs. K. Shimamoto, E. Domino, M. Seevers, E. Carr, Jr., T. Brody.
Row 2 from left: Drs. B. Lucchesi, T. Yanagita, L. Beck, E. Cafruny, D. Bennett, L. Mellett, H. Swain.
Row 3 from left: Drs. S. Takaori, R. Reynolds, S. Kayaalp, J. Magana, P. Saxena, P. Chipps, G. Deneau.

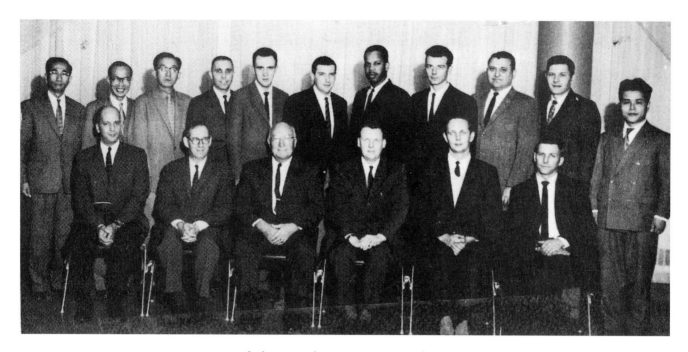

Department of Pharmacology, University of Michigan, 1962.
Row 1 from left: Drs. E. Cafruny, T. Brody, M. Seevers, E. Carr, Jr., H. Swain, L. Beck.
Row 2 from left: Drs. S. Hisada, S. Iida, T. Furukawa, B. Lucchesi, J. Villarreal, M. Segal, R. Hudson,
G. Deneau, B. Mellett, D. Bennett, T. Yanagita.

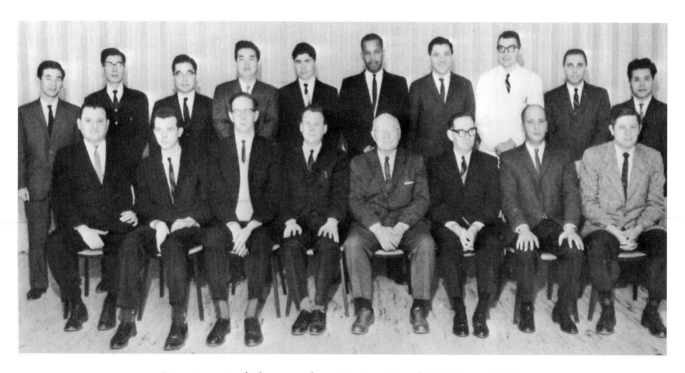

Department of Pharmacology, University of Michigan, 1964.
Row 1 from left: Drs. B. Mellett, G. Deneau, H. Swain, E. Carr, Jr., M.H. Seevers, T. Brody, E. Cafruny,
D. Bennett.
Row 2 from left: Drs. R. Inoki, N. Katsuda, T. Akera, K. Yamamoto, Unidentified, Drs. R. Hudson,
C. Schuster, W. Baird, B. Lucchesi, T. Yanagita.

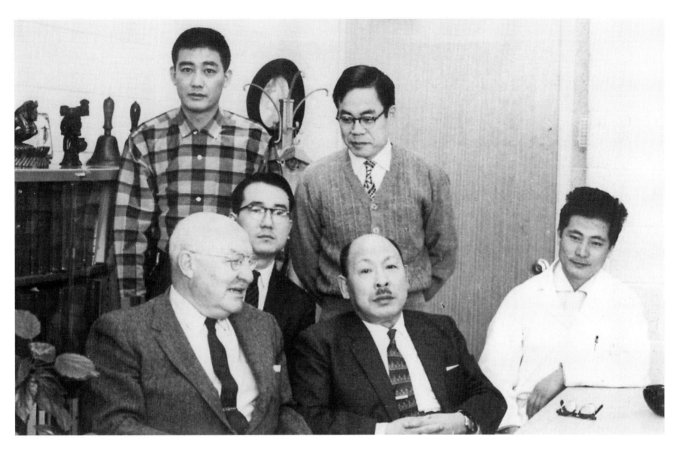

Fellows meeting in Dr. Seevers' office in the Department of Pharmacology, Ann Arbor, 1960.
Row 1 from left: Drs. M.H. Seevers, S. Takaori, Unidentified, Dr. H. Kaneto.
Row 2 from left: Drs. A. Sakuma, K. Nakai.

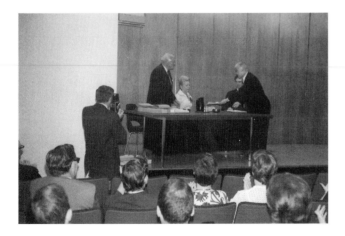

Dr. Seevers' retirement symposium, May 28, 1970, Ann Arbor.

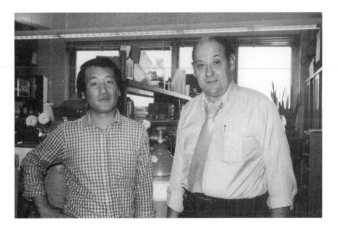

Drs. N. Fukuda and E.F. Domino in laboratory in Ann Arbor, 1981.

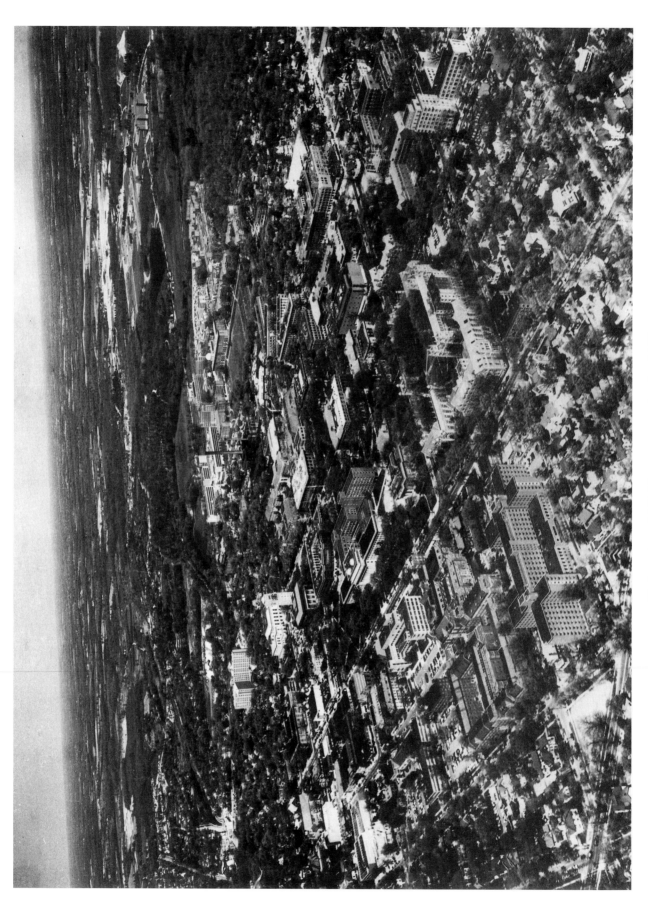

University of Michigan campus in the 1960s.

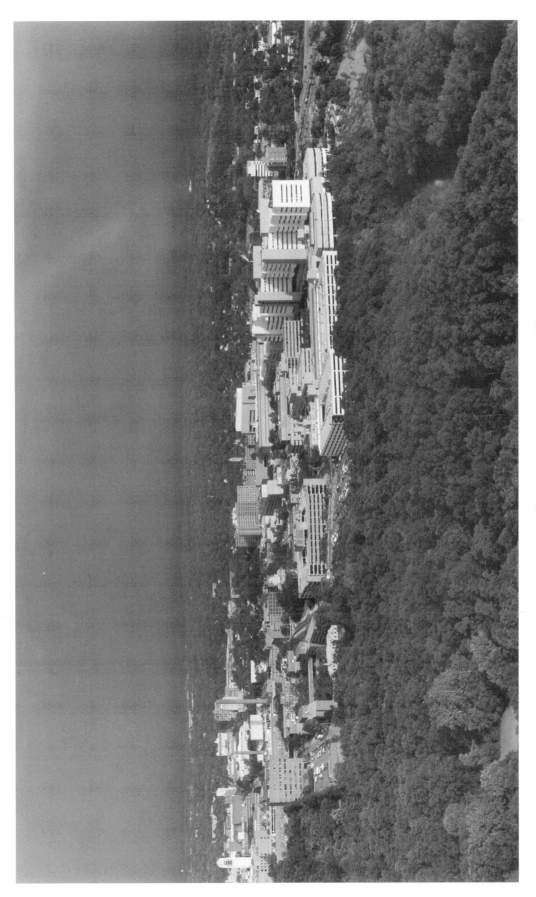

University of Michigan campus in the 1980s.

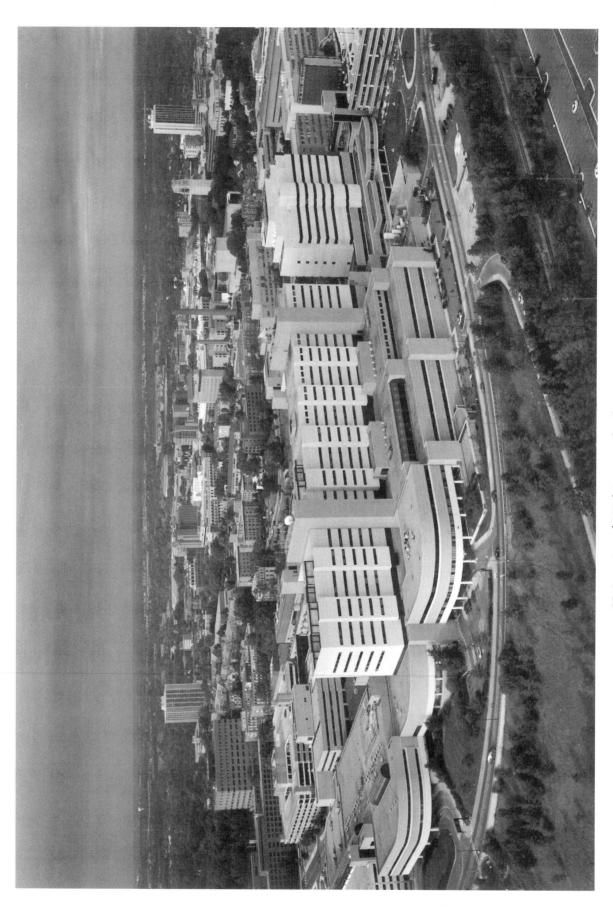

University of Michigan Medical Center in 1997.

Appendix B5. Some Japanese Michigan Fellows

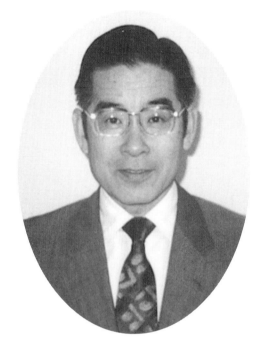

Dr. T. Akera

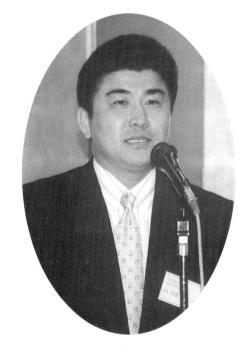

Dr. T. Endo

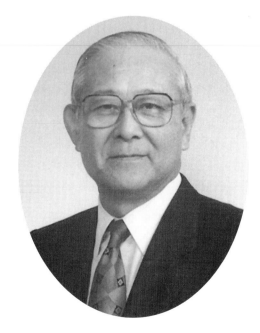

Dr. T. Fukuda

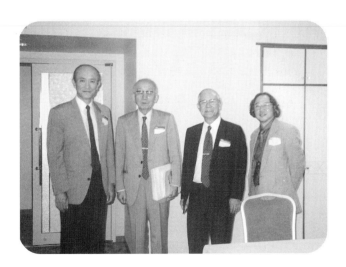

Dr. T. Fukuda with Michigan Fellows
Dr. T. Furukawa and Dr. T. Yamamoto and
colleague.

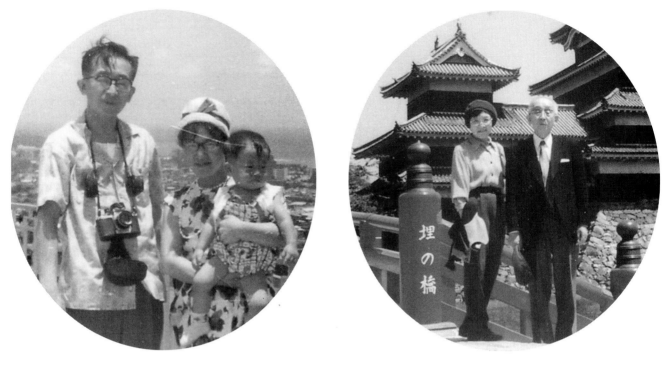

Dr. and Mrs. T. Furukawa then and now.

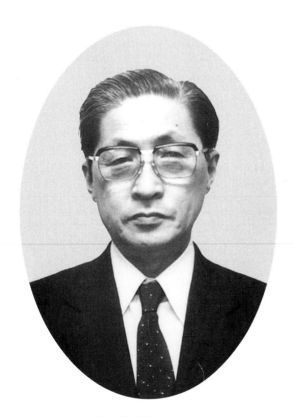

Dr. E. Hasegawa

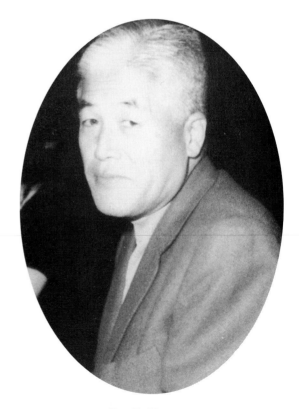

Dr. E. Hosoya

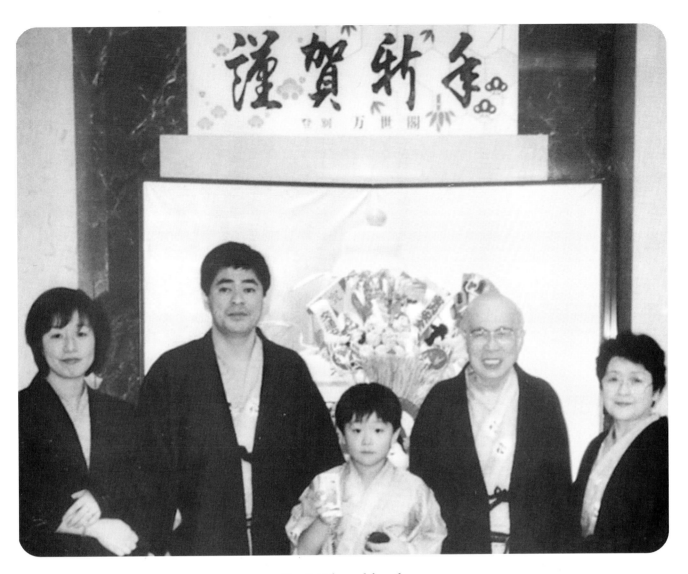

Dr. S. Iida and family

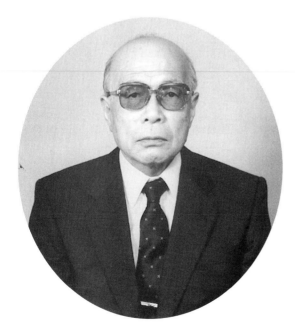

Dr. S. Iida

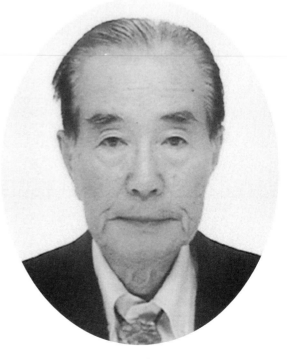

Dr. F. Ikomi

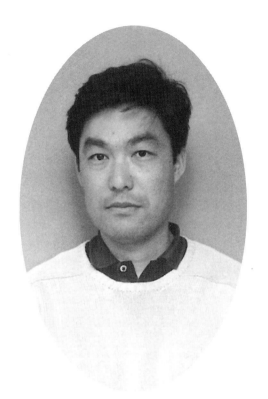

Dr. S. Iwata

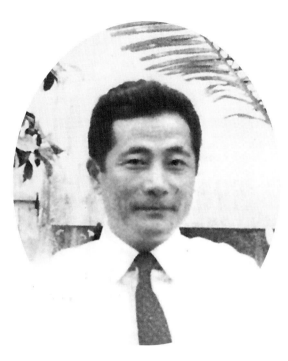

Dr. H. Kaneto

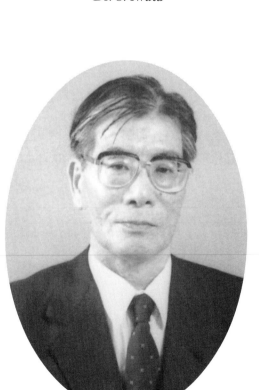

Dr. N. Katsuda

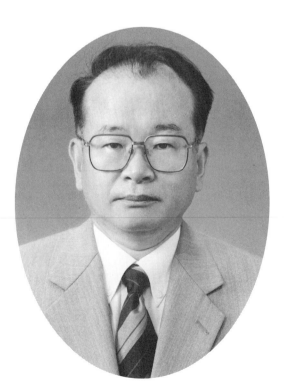

Dr. M. Minami

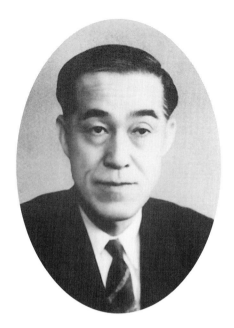

Dr. T. Murano

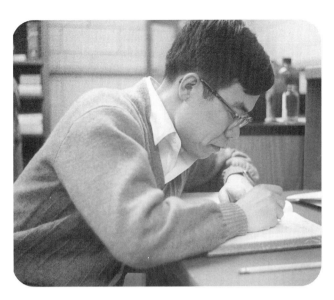

Dr. K. Nakai

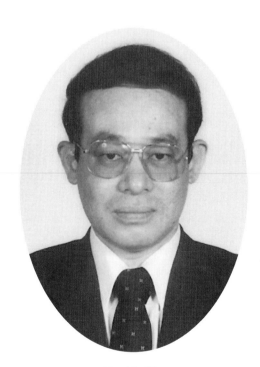

Dr. T. Oka

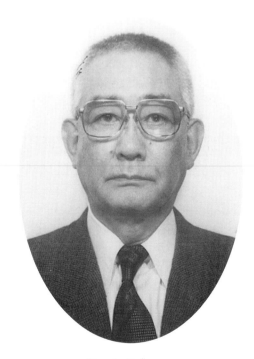

Dr. A. Sakuma

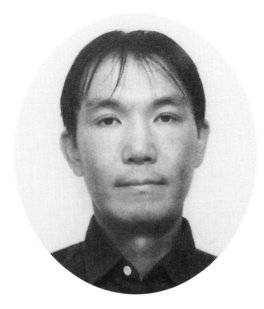

Dr. Y. Sudo

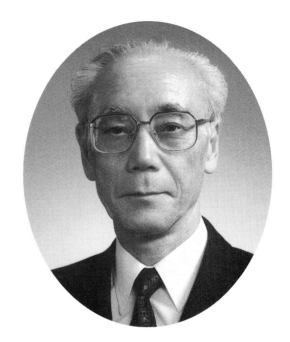

Dr. S. Tadokoro

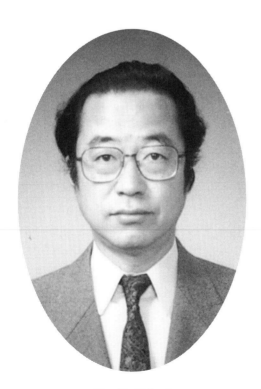

Dr. K. Takada

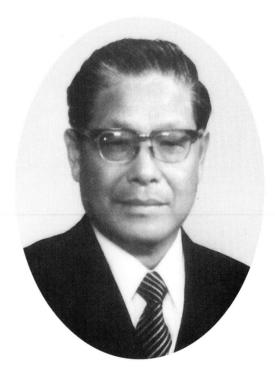

Dr. T. Tanabe

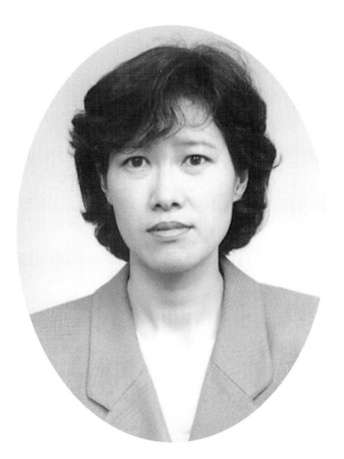

Dr. H. Togashi

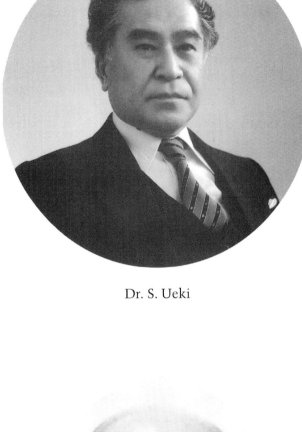

Dr. S. Ueki

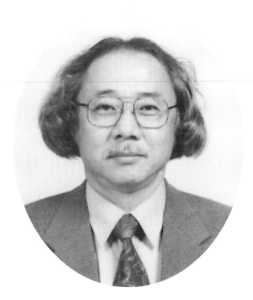

Dr. T. Yamamoto

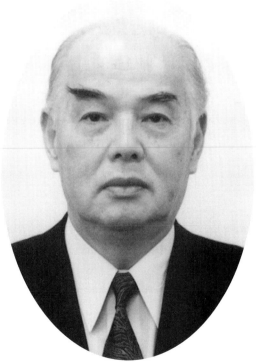

Dr. K. Yamamoto

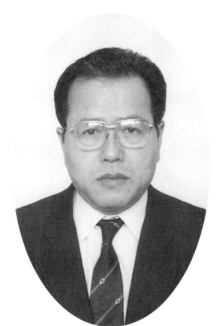

Dr. T. Yanagita

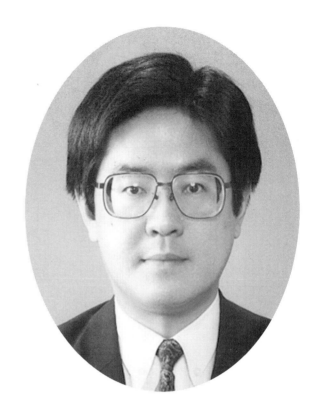

Dr. M. Yoshioka

MICHIGAN
WOLVERINES

Appendix C: History of The Seevers' Bonsai Tree Collection at Matthaei Botanical Gardens

Connie C. Bailie, B.S.

For the past 10 years, I have been a horticultural assistant at the Matthaei Botanical Gardens. From 1989–1991, I also worked as a volunteer to take care of the Seevers' bonsai trees. In 1991, I was given the responsibility for their care as part of my horticultural duties. Over the years, various volunteers of the Ann Arbor Bonsai Society, of which Dr. Seevers was a founding member, have also been involved in the care and maintenance of the bonsai collection.

The bonsai collection started in 1977 with the donation of Dr. Seevers' trees by his wife, Frances, soon after his death. At that time, the gardens were undergoing severe financial cutbacks. The donation of such a labor intensive collection was received with some trepidation. To offset the cost of maintaining the collection, a number of bonsai from the collection were sold, mostly to members of the Ann Arbor Bonsai Society.

During the first five years, the collection floundered somewhat under the care of staff not experienced with bonsai. Daily horticultural needs, so vitally important with such a demanding collection, were not consistent, nor were styling efforts. It was not until the arrival of staff familiar with bonsai that the collection received the horticultural care that it required. Soon after, the Director of the Gardens asked the members of the Ann Arbor Bonsai Society to become more actively involved. They evaluated and gave recommendations for the future care and styling of the 17 remaining trees. The Ann Arbor Bonsai Society remains an integral part of the upkeep of the collection. Four of the best specimens are shown in the figures on the following pages.

The collection grew handsomely, health returned, and pruning was administered regularly. The trees developed to become one of our prized collections. Through the years, volunteers who were mostly members of the Ann Arbor Bonsai Society, have come and gone. Each volunteer has added tremendously to the overall health and appeal of the collection. It has been the good fortune of the Gardens to have such capable participation in the upkeep of the collection. However, styling goals were inconsistent some years. Of late, consistency of training has again become important, as well as detailed record keeping. Area experts are called on to consult yearly as to the goals of the current growing season.

Unfortunately, although the Seevers' bonsai had grown, flourished, and become dramatic, each in its own way, the collection had not become an integral part of our public displays. The problem of developing an area which could be secure and aesthetic was not settled until this year, 1998, 21 years after the collection was received. We are proud to announce that the Seevers' collection, along with other newly obtained tropical bonsai, will now be part of a rotating display in the warm temperature house of our public conservatory.

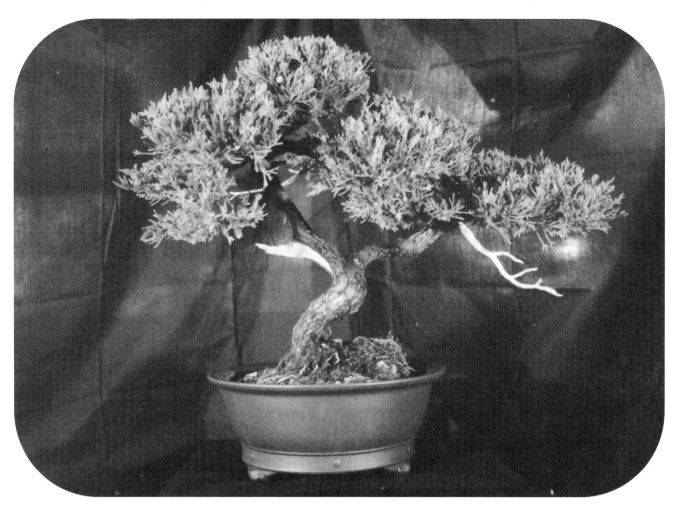

Fig. 1. *Juniper* species. Wind swept style. Photograph taken October 14, 1996.

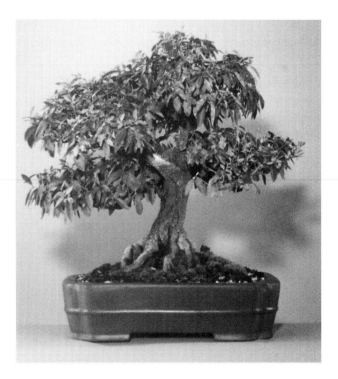

Fig. 2. *Ligustrum* species. Informal upright style. Photograph taken in 1997.

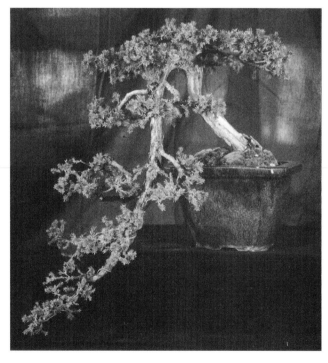

Fig. 3. *Juniper procumbens* "Nana." Cascade style. Photograph taken October 14, 1996.

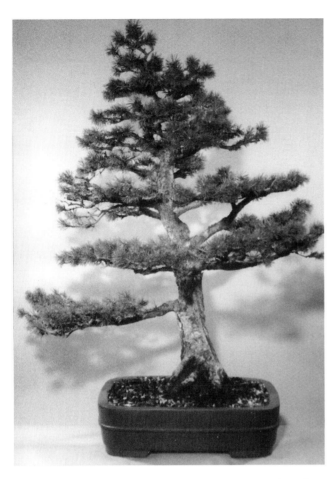

Fig. 4. *Pinus sylvestris.* Informal upright style. Photograph taken October 26, 1997.

The warm temperature house is undergoing a major reworking. The entire room was gutted and new hardscape installed. What was once simply a plant diversity plan for biology students is now redesigned as an area to display an interesting and diverse group of plants in the context of cultural aspects. As part of this new plan, an Asian area will be incorporated and will give us an opportunity to display all of the bonsai, including the Seevers' collection, in an interesting fashion year round.

The Seevers' collection is mostly comprised of hardy, traditional plant material that needs a cooling temperature each winter to satisfy the chilling factor of each tree in order to resume growth in the spring. During the first week of November, the Seevers' trees are put in a deep coldframe to overwinter to avoid subzero freezing of the roots. Because of their seasonality, display of the trees is limited to the growing season from April to November. During this time, the glasshouse environment limits sunlight and fresh air. The trees will only be displayed for one week at a time, returning to an outside bench to rejuvenate. While the hardy material is overwintering the tropical bonsai will be displayed in the Asian area. Therefore, the conservatory bonsai display will change regularly, giving incentive for visitors to revisit the display and view a changing array of trees and styles.

We especially invite the Japanese Michigan Fellows in Pharmacology, their families, and friends to visit the Gardens and view this collection as a reminder of the impact of Japan here in Ann Arbor, Michigan.

Epilogue

————◀○▶————

It was impossible for us to identify all of the activities and contributions of the Japanese Michigan fellows. We apologize for anyone we have unintentionally omitted or for any facts we have wrong. As can be seen from the enclosed, the impact of Japanese Michigan fellows upon Japanese society, through medical and pharmaceutical education, research, and public service, has been and continues to be profound. We are pleased that the efforts and courtesy of Dr. Seevers and the Department of Pharmacology at the University of Michigan in welcoming and training Japanese postdoctoral fellows have been fruitful. All the Michigan fellows are very thankful for and proud of having had the opportunity to study at Michigan. From the department's side, the Japanese postdoctoral fellows proved to be very productive and stimulating in maintaining departmental activities. So, what else is there to say but "let's continue." We, both at Michigan and in Japan, should make further efforts to assure the continuation of this wonderful tradition for a long time into the future.

Tomoji Yanagita
Edward F. Domino

Index of Japanese Michigan Fellows, Colleagues, and Friends

Bold number indicates the page of a biographical sketch.